The Advanced Practitioner

Current Practice Issues

Joellen W. Hawkins, RNC, Ph.D., FAAN
Professor, Boston College
Janice A. Thibodeau, RN,C, Ed.D., FAAN
Professor, University of Connecticut

Third Edition

The Tiresias Press, Inc., New York

Dedication

To Andrew, Dana, David, Gillian, Glen, John, Marshall, Lillian Beck Fuller, R.N., and our parents.

Copyright ® 1993
The Tiresias Press, Inc.
116 Pinehurst Avenue, New York, NY 10033
All Right Reserved

Library of Congress
Catalog Card Number: 93-060215
International Standard
Book Number: 0-913292-38-9

Printed in U.S.A.

The Advanced Practitioner

Current Practice Issues

Contents

Preface, 7

1. Using a Nursing Model for Advanced Practice, 9
2. Advanced Practice Roles: Nurse Practitioner/Clinical Nurse Specialist, 18
3. Effects of Sex-Role Stereotyping on Leadership in Nursing: Need for a Feminist Paradigm, 42
4. Power and Nursing: Need for a Paradigm of Empowerment, 52
5. The Concept of Change, 62
6. Legal Aspects of Advanced Practice Roles, 72
7. Continuous Quality Improvement, 87
8. The Role of Research in Advanced Practice, 112
9. Negotiating an Employment Contract, 130
10. Economics of the Roles, 141
11. Mentorship, 163
12. Community Assessment, 174

Appendices
A. Scope of Practice Statements and Role Definitions, 189
B. Resources on Legal and Ethical Aspects, Credentialing, and Certification, 190
C. Evaluation Tool for Primary Care with Children, 192
D. Evaluation Tool for Primary Care with Older Adults, 195
E. Funding Sources. Publications, 198
F. Sources for Information on Grants, 199
G. Research References, 200

Index, 201

Acknowledgments

To our students over many years, whose feedback has been invaluable in the development of material for this book, we owe many thanks. Our colleagues in practice have added their support and input as this book evolved.

We are especially grateful to Catherine Collins for allowing us to use the evaluation tools she developed for her practice.

Most of all, we owe our deepest gratitude to our friends and families for their support of us and tolerance of our seemingly endless projects.

Joellen W. Hawkins
Janice A. Thibodeau

ABOUT THE AUTHORS

Joellen W. Hawkins is a professor at Boston College and a certified obstetrical/gynecological nurse practitioner. Her many books include *Nursing and the American Health Care Delivery System, The Dictionary of American Nursing Biography,* and *Protocols for Nurse Practitioners in Gynecologic Settings.*

Janice A. Thibodeau is a professor at the University of Connecticut and a certified adult nurse practitioner. She is the author of *Nursing Models: Analysis and Evaluation.*

Preface

This book is intended to be a text for students enrolled in advanced practice programs and as a reference for nurses who are already advanced practitioners. It translates broad, theoretical concepts into the practical, everyday concerns of nurses in advanced practice roles, and, by analyzing selected issues affecting role implementation, it directs students and nurses already active as advanced practitioners to assume, examine, and reality test the various aspects of these roles.

The issues addressed here are those concerned with aspects of being an advanced practitioner beyond the care of clients: negotiating for a job; credentialing for advanced practice; economics of health care delivery; legal aspects of practice; scope of practice; use of a nursing model for practice; use of change theory; concepts of power, authority, leadership, and sex-role stereotyping; research in advanced practice roles; quality improvement for practice; communication and assertiveness; mentoring; and community assessment for improved or expanded delivery of care by nurses.

1
Using a Nursing Model for Advanced Practice

Introduction

This is a text designed for advanced practitioners who practice in all health care settings and for graduate students who are learning the advanced practice roles. The role of the advanced practitioner is multifaceted, complex and diversified.

Advanced Practice

Inherent in the role of an advanced practitioner is accountability and responsibility for decisions made and actions rendered. This responsibility is retained even when a referral to another health care provider is indicated. By using a nursing model as a guide, the nurse practitioner or clinical nurse specialist can assess the supports and constraints within the system and plan care accordingly. Constraints can be identified and strategies can be developed to overcome them. Supports can be mobilized to provide high quality nursing care.

Nursing Models

A nursing model provides detailed guidelines for organizing and collecting data for planning and implementing management and change strategies and evaluating total role functions. A model defines the essence and boundaries of the care rendered as well as explicitly stating the role of the nurse and the client. Delineating boundaries is especially important in light of the legal ramifications associated with advanced practice and expanded role function. A nursing model also specifies the ultimate goal of the nursing process. This is an important aspect to clarify because the ultimate goal of the nursing process, as dictated by one's model of practice, may differ from that of the agency employing the practitioner or clinical specialist. This discrepancy can lead to basic philosophical differences which can cause role conflict and confusion. A nursing model helps to bring the often nebulous philosophical issues into sharper focus.

At the present time, there are many models of nursing practice in various stages of development. Among these are the Crisis Model, the Rogers Life Process Model, the Roy Adaptation Model, Orem's Self Care Model, and the Neuman Health Care Systems Model. Caring is the focus of a number of contemporary models. Among these are those of Benner and Wrubel, Leininger, and Watson. The advanced practitioner must think carefully about her/his philosophies of nursing and health care and about the relationships between these two belief systems. Since one's philosophy is derived from one's cultural and social experiences, there is no right or wrong philosophy. One must honestly strive to know what one believes about nursing and its practice so that a model of practice can be chosen that is compatible with these beliefs. Thibodeau's *Nursing Models: Analysis and Evaluation* gives specific guidelines for selecting and evaluating a model of practice (1).

Advanced clinical practice and expanded nursing role functions should be guided by a nursing model and not by the medical model. Nursing management of clients, client advocacy, improvement of methods of health care delivery, and broad health assessment and planning are integral components of nursing's role. These functions are not extensions of medicine, nor do they fall within the framework of medical protocols. In education, practice, and research, nursing has clearly been moving away from the medical model approach to health care delivery. A study by Thibodeau and Hawkins (2) found that advanced practitioners see themselves as nurses with a broader focus than that inherent in the medical paradigm. These nurses have strong images of themselves in their roles through their strong orientation toward a nursing model. Early practitioner programs were directed or codirected by physicians. As a result, there has always been the danger of practicing according to the medical rather than a nursing model in the nurse's delivery of primary care. Incorporating physical assessment and history-taking skills into one's practice does not have to lead to junior doctoring. Nurses and physicians should complement each other because their assessment skills are utilized for different ends. The acute care setting, with its history of medical dominance, holds the same danger for the clinical nurse specialist of being co-opted by the medical model.

The lure of following the medical model is sanctioned and well rewarded in some settings. Johnson (3) states that a number of nurses have chosen the medical model of practice because they do not think nursing has a destiny of its own or because they believe their identity depends on the sanction of physicians. Some nurses may feel that the medical model offers them greater challenges and responsibilities - until they realize that nurses can never have freedom and autonomy using that model.

The medical model focuses on signs, symptoms, pathology, prognoses, and the course of disease. This disease-oriented approach attends to the structure and functions of the body rather than to the total person. It ignores the environment and the psychosocial factors that surround illness, including quality of life and ethics (4). "The medical model posits a dichotomy between mind and body which is not congruent with the philosophy of nursing in its concerns with the whole person. Not only is nursing concerned with the structure and function of the body; it is also concerned with human experience, behavior, feelings, and the influence of social forces upon the body — manifestations of the man-environment interaction" (5). The nurse's expanded role and advanced clinical practice should not have a medical orientation. Since assessment skills are used as adjuncts to the nursing process, their incorporation into the nursing role is best done within the context of a conceptual model of nursing practice.

What is the essence of nursing, its boundaries, and its goals? Although there is still much discussion as to the nature of nursing, there is basic agreement within the profession as to the four essential concepts of a nursing model. These are: person, environment, health, and nursing. Other disciplines may address one, two, or even three of these concepts, but all four elements must be addressed if a model is to be considered a nursing model.

Person. A nursing model must describe the nature of the person. The individual may be seen as an active or passive being who cooperates with the environment, controls the environment, or is controlled by it.

The wholeness and integrity of the individual may be emphasized, or emphasis may be placed on individual, unique attributes. Equal attention may be placed on the physical, spiritual, social, cultural, and psychological aspects of the individual's nature, or some aspects of the person may receive undue attention to the exclusion of other aspects. The nature of the person influences very directly the nature of nursing.

Environment. Environment can be viewed as all of the influences and circumstances surrounding and affecting people. Environment has both an internal and an external component. The internal environment relates to factors such as personality, mental capacity, and genetic make-up. The external environment includes all factors outside the individual. The nurse is part of the individual's external environment. It is evident that the nature of person-environment interactions as described by a given model also greatly influences the nature of nursing.

Health. Health and illness may be conceptualized on a continuum as co-existent states or mutually exclusive states (see Figure 1.1). Health may be viewed as a behavior or from a physical, mental or social perspective. A physical perspective emphasizes observable and measurable manifestations of illness. A mental perspective emphasizes the person's state of mind, that is, how the individual feels. A social perspective emphasizes disruptions in activities of daily living or inability to carry out prescribed roles, such as that of parent or worker. Health-illness is described in any given nursing model. Since one of the goals of nursing is to promote health, it is evident how the perception of health directly influences the practice of nursing. Knutson (6) suggests that the evolution from a medical to a nursing model has changed the focus of our practices from illness care to health care.

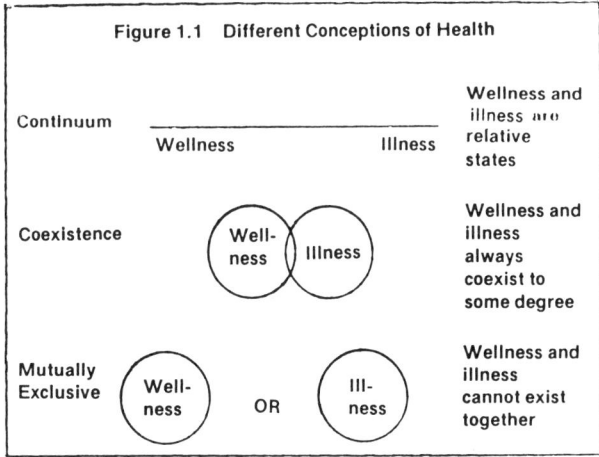

Nursing. Nursing models speak specifically to the nature of nursing, its goals, and the process utilized to achieve these goals. The role of the nurse is implicitly or explicitly addressed in any given nursing model.

At the present time, there is no dominant model for nursing that clearly and explicitly guides the majority of practitioners of nursing. Nor does one model set the direction for all nursing education and research endeavors. Today, any nursing model only dictates that the four essential components of nursing's metaparadigm (person, health, environment, and nursing) be addressed. A nursing model describes how each of these elements is precisely defined and depicted. By doing so, it focuses thinking in a particular way. Wilbur (7) suggests that practitioners are developing their own theoretical frameworks out of their practice experiences. A model outlines nursing practice in a way that can be reality tested and corroborated. Nursing models are devices by which assumptions held by nurses about their practice can be transformed into postulates which can be tested through research.

A model generates researchable questions which, if answered by a process of scientific inquiry, lead to the development of nursing theory. This theory would truly belong to the field of nursing and could be described as unique rather than borrowed theory. Johnson describes borrowed theory as knowledge which is developed by other disciplines and which is then drawn upon by nursing. Unique theory is that knowledge which is derived from generation to generation of hypotheses unlike those that characterize other disciplines (8). A nursing model is the direct pathway to nursing theory.

Use of a Nursing Model in Advanced Practice

A model directly guides nursing management of clients in all health care settings. It guides the collection of data, the planning of care, the implementation of care, and the evaluation of that care. Since the model outlines the boundaries and essence of the discipline, practice of a given model is directly related to the scope of practice statements which are discussed in Chapter Two.

Being able to practice according to one's conceptual nursing model may be difficult in many medically-oriented settings. Therefore, putting one's model into practice requires a thorough knowledge of the concepts of power, politics, and leadership which are discussed in Chapter Three. Using assertive techniques can also be helpful in actualizing one's model. Strategies to help the practitioner and clinical specialist become more assertive are discussed in Chapter Four.

Since a model lends direction to practice, the advanced practitioner must be a change agent who understands the theory and process of change. The boundaries and essence of practice are influenced by legal ramifications and nurse practice acts. These concepts are discussed in Chapters Five and Six.

Using a model to guide nursing management results in standardizing care, making it easier to collect data for research. By facilitating the research process, the advanced practitioner is assisted in developing a prescriptive theory to guide clinical practice and improve the quality of care rendered. Quality improvement and nursing research are discussed in Chapters Seven and Eight. Chapter Nine focuses on the practical aspects of using a nursing philosophy to guide the process of negotiating an employment contract, and Chapter Ten continues with a discussion of the economics of practice. Chapter Eleven focuses on career development and advancement, with a specific emphasis on mentorship. The closing chapter, Chapter Twelve, discusses the role of the advanced practitioner in improving health by conducting community ssessments.

Summary

A nursing model provides guidelines for the role functions of advanced practitioners. The philosophy of the practitioner determines her or his choice of a model of nursing practice. A model is a description of the concepts of person, environment, health, and nursing and of the interrelationships among these concepts. A model outlines nursing practice in a way that can be reality tested and corroborated. It guides the collection of data, the planning of care, the implementation of care, and the evaluation of care. One's model of practice has implications for all areas of role function, including standards of practice, legal aspects of practice, and quality improvement.

REFERENCES

1. Thibodeau, J. (1983). Nursing Models: Analysis and Evaluation. Monterey, CA: Wadsworth.

2. Thibodeau, J. & Hawkins, J. (1992). Moving toward a nursing model in advanced practice. Funded by Mu Chapter, Sigma Theta Tau.
3. Johnson, P.E. (1974). Development of theory: A requisite for nursing as a primary health profession. Nursing Research 23:372-377.
4. Allen, J. & Hall, B. (1988). Changing the focus on technology: A critique of the medical model in the health care system. Advances in Nursing Science 10:22-35.
5. Phillips, J.R. (1977). Nursing systems and nursing models. Image 9:4-7.
6. Knutson, K. (1990). 25 years later: 25 exceptional NPs look at the movement's evolution and consider future challenges for the role. The Nurse Practitioner 15:20.
7. Wilbur, J. (1990). 25 years later: 25 exceptional NPs look at the movement's evolution and consider future challenges for the role. The Nurse Practitioner 15:14.
8. Johnson, P.E. (1968). Theory in nursing: Borrowed and unique. Nursing Research 17:206-209.

BIBLIOGRAPHY

Andrews, H.A. & Roy, C. (1986). Essentials of the Roy Adaptation Model. Norwalk, CT: Appleton-Century-Crofts.
Benner, P. & Wrubel, J. (1989). The Primacy of Caring. Menlo Park, CA: Addison-Wesley.
Buchanan, B. (1987). Conceptual models: An assessment framework. Journal of Nursing Administration 17:22-26.
Fawcett, J. (1984). Analysis and Evaluation of Conceptual Models of Nursing. Philadelphia: F.A. Davis.
Jennings, B. & Meleis, A. (1988). Nursing theory and administrative practice: Agenda for the 1990's. Advances in Nursing Science 10:56-70.
Leininger, M. (1988). Caring. The Proceedings of the National Caring

Conferences. Detroit: Wayne State Press.
Marriner, A. (1986). Nursing Theorists and Their Work. St. Louis, MO: C.V. Mosby.
Neuman, B. (1988). The Neuman Systems Model. Norwalk, CT: Appleton & Lange.
Orem, D.E. (1985). Concepts of Practice. 3rd ed. New York: McGraw-Hill.
Rogers, M. (1985). An Introduction to the Theoretical Basis of Nursing. Philadelphia: F.A. Davis.
Sarter, B. (1988). The Stream of Becoming. A Study of Martha Rogers' Theory. New York: National League for Nursing (Pub. #15-2205).
Watson, J. (1985). Nursing: Human Science and Human Care. New York: Appleton-Century Crofts.

2
Advanced Practice Roles: Nurse Practitioner/Clinical Nurse Specialist

Introduction

The concept of an expanding role for nurses embodied in the nurse practitioner and clinical nurse specialist movements is not new. Ford (1) cites the examples of Florence Nightingale and Lillian Wald. Both of these nurses — Nightingale in the Crimea and later in her astute planning for nursing practice and education, and Wald in the tenements of New York City — reflected a scope of practice akin to that of today's "new" practitioners. Ford also notes that Esther Lucile Brown (2) called for an expansion of the role of nurses in research. Mary Breckinridge, in founding the Frontier Nursing Service, demonstrated the value of nurses as primary care providers in the hills of Kentucky (3). Thus, the concept is not unique to the later decades of the twentieth century, although it has, in the years since 1965, acquired titles and more formal definitions.

Historical Evolution

The first nurse practitioner demonstration project, in 1965, was planned to "determine the safety, efficacy, and quality of a new mode of nursing practice designed to improve health care to children and families and to develop a new nursing role - that of the pediatric nurse practitioner" (4). Loretta Ford was codirector of the project, which took place at the University of Colorado. Frances Reiter first used the term nurse-clinician in a 1943 speech. In 1944, Adelaide A. Mayo defined the clinical nurse specialist in an article in the *American Journal of Nursing* (5). Dorothy Johnson offered clinical nurse specialists as a solution to the problem of the well-prepared nurse moving away from direct patient care (6). An early master's program to prepare advanced practitioners was developed by Hildegard Peplau at Rutgers University in 1954. It focused on psychiatric nursing (7). Two years later, at an interdisciplinary conference, participants agreed that clinical specialists in psychiatric nursing should be prepared at the master's level (8).

Nurse practitioner and clinical nurse specialist programs were given a boost by the Nurse Training Act of 1964 (PL 88-581), Title II of the 1968 Health Manpower Act (PL 92-158), and the Nurse Training Act of 1975 (PL 94-63). All of these provided monies for advanced nurse training and the establishment of practitioner programs (9)

In 1971, the Committee of the Secretary of Health, Education, and Welfare presented its findings from a study of extended roles for nurses. The report concluded that nurses can assume responsibility for extended roles in primary care, in acute care, and in long-term care; in some cases with additional preparation.

Also in 1971, the University of Washington began a program to prepare family nurse practitioners. Following that example, which became known as PRIMEX, programs were initiated at Cornell-New York Hospital and the University of North Carolina at Chapel Hill (10). Other early programs included the family nurse practitioner program at the University of California, Davis; Boston College's programs in ambulatory care for women and children which were piloted in 1967 and funded by the Macy Foundation in 1968; and the program at Wayne State for health nurse clinicians (11).

Recognizing the need for a statement from the professional nursing organization on the expanded role, in 1974 the ANA Congress of Nursing Practice published definitions of the advanced practice roles. These definitions not only addressed matters of the scope of practice but, in addition, stated that skills are to be acquired in continuing education programs following ANA guidelines or in baccalaureate nursing programs (12).

In the late 1960s, certification and examinations were developed by the ANA Divisions of Practice. Among the first nurses certified with advanced practice degrees were those in psychiatric mental health practice (13). Then, in 1976, an ANA program was implemented to provide for certification of nurses as nurse practitioners (14). Thus, in a little over two decades from the first formal nurse practitioner and clinical nurse specialist programs, the concept of role expansion for nurses took hold and gave birth to new definitions of practice and the process of credentialing for advanced practice.

In a longitudinal study of nurse practitioners, 87 certificate and 46 master's degree programs were identified in approximately 100 institutions. All of these programs had begun prior to 1974 (15). In the 1973-74 directory of programs preparing nurses for expanded roles, 83 certificate programs are listed, ranging in length from three-quarters of a month to two years. This list includes certificate programs preparing nurse midwives. The same directory lists 21 schools awarding a master's degree, 13 of which list nurse midwifery and/or nurse practitioner as role options. These programs range in length from one to two years (16). In 1979, it was estimated that there were approximately 198 nurse practitioner programs producing 1,800 graduates a year. The majority of the programs remained certificate (124) as compared with 74 granting a master's degree (17). By 1990, there were 84 master's programs offering one or more nurse practitioner options and 11 certificate programs (18, 19). In the core curriculum survey, 122 programs offering master's preparation in one or more nurse practitioner specialty areas were identified (20). Some of these are combined nurse practitioner/clinical nurse specialist programs.

Adding to the confusion is the lack of unity in requirements for entry into nurse practitioner programs. Many of the certificate programs require only that one be a registered nurse with a current license to practice. Admission requirements range from physician recommendation and a promise to serve as preceptor to meeting criteria for admission to the graduate school of a university (7). Upon completion, the individual may receive nothing, a certificate, a baccalaureate degree, or master's degree (7). Settings for programs range from physician's offices to hospitals, other health care institutions, schools of nursing, universities and colleges, and schools of public health and medicine. The debate continues concerning the setting for and length of practitioner programs. Federal guidelines mandate that programs be one year in length in order to qualify for funding. Guidelines for programs have been prepared by the American Nurses Association, the Association of Women's Health, Obstetric, and Neonatal Nurses, the American College of Nurse Midwives, and the National Association of Pediatric Nurse Associates and Practitioners. Graduates of programs adhering to the guidelines are eligible for certification examinations sponsored by these organizations (see this chapter's Bibliography for a list of guidelines).

In 1979, the National League for Nursing published a position paper on the education of nurse practitioners, stating that "the nurse practitioner should hold a master's degree in nursing in order to ensure competence and quality care." The statement then emphasized the need for nurses to be educated as practitioners within the formal structure of graduate nursing programs (21). More than a decade later, nurse practitioners do not need to hold a baccalaureate degree to practice in many states (22). In 1993, preparation at the graduate level is required to sit for certification examinations offered by the American Nurses Credentialing Center as an adult, family, pediatric, school, or gerontologic nurse practitioner, and by 1998 all generalist certification examinations will require a minimum of a baccalaureate degree (23).

Educational preparation for clinical nurse specialists/nurse clinicians evolved in a somewhat different model from that for nurse practitioners. Beginning in 1954, master's programs were developed whose focus was advanced clinical practice (7). Unlike the deluge of programs to prepare nurse practitioners, no comparable explosion of certificate programs occurred to prepare clinical nurse specialists. Most, if not all, of the programs were at the master's level. By 1990, NLN listed 231 master's programs offering preparation in one or more specialty areas for clinical nurse specialists and/or other advanced practice roles (24). The results of the clinical nurse specialist and nurse practitioner core curricula survey demonstrate that at the master's level, preparation for both roles is quite similar. Differences exist in clinical content (pharmacology, primary care, history taking and physical assessment, nutrition, and health promotion in nurse practitioner programs and in clinical settings (with more secondary and tertiary for clinical specialists) (25).

Advanced Practice Roles: Blending and Merging

By the mid 1980s, the differences between nurse practitioners and clinical nurse specialists were blurring. Certificate practitioner programs were declining and the number of master's programs were rising (26). In a working document for the Council of Clinical Nurse Specialists and the Council of Primary Care Nurse Practitioners of the American Nurses Association, Sparacino and Durand laid out the similarities and differences in the two advanced practice roles (27). In 1990, the two councils merged, reflecting a transition to designation as nurses in advanced practice (28, 29).

Of course, such a merger does not occur without dissent. Some have argued that clinical specialists should move toward the nurse practitioner name and role, in part because of the power base and public recognition associated with the title nurse practitioner (30). In several studies, merging of roles is evident. Edler and Bullough (31) surveyed graduates of nurse practitioner and clinical nurse specialist programs and found fewer differences than the literature might suggest and a general consensus that the roles should merge. The core curriculum study supports congruence in master's preparation between the two roles, as noted earlier (19). Diers (32) argues that we no longer have "generalized practice." Advanced nurse practitioners should be prepared for specialty practice at the master's level (33). The greatest differentiation between clinical nurse specialists and nurse practitioners occurred as education programs developed on divergent paths: certificate and master's. With convergence of those paths, merging of the roles becomes clearer.

Practice Settings

When Lucille Kinlein became an independent practitioner over a decade ago, she was declaring to the public that she, as a nurse, had something unique and special to offer to clients (34). Numerous other nurses have followed her example and have met with varied success (35). Jacox and Norris (36) have collected the report of a conference held in 1975. This document explores problems and issues confronting nurses who go into private and independent practice.

Settings for practice vary widely among those nurses calling themselves and practicing as nurse practitioners and as clinical nurse specialists.

By 1988, 23,000 nurse practitioners, 4,200 nurse-midwives, and more than 30,000 clinical nurse specialists were employed in the U.S. Practice settings included hospitals (federal, psychiatric, tuberculosis, long- and short-term general), nursing homes, schools of nursing, public health agencies, college and university student health services, public and private schools, early intervention programs, nursing homes, senior centers, work sites, prisons, ambulatory care agencies, and self-employment (15). Clinical nurse specialists were employed in the same settings, but in differing proportions, particularly those holding positions in hospitals (37). Psychiatric nurses with a master's degree or above, in many cases indicating clinical specialization in psychiatric-mental health nursing, are employed in outpatient facilities, state and county hospitals, private psychiatric hospitals, residential treatment centers for emotionally disturbed children, other types of residential facilities, VA psychiatric organizations, mental health partial care organizations, and multiservice mental health organizations (15). The 1980s added yet another type of setting for nurses with advanced practice preparation: shelters for the homeless, for battered women, and soup kitchens (38).

A number of authors have suggested that nurse practitioners and clinical nurse specialists must learn to market themselves to potential clients. Some of their articles focus on the role of advanced practitioners in private practice, others on new or enlarging client groups such as older adults, or in nontraditional settings such as ambulatory centers managed by other than physicians (39, 40, 41, 42). Towers (43) reported from a national survey of nurse practitioners that fewer than half of the respondents market themselves. When they do, they use pamphlets, the yellow pages, newspaper ads, and special referral arrangements. Hershey (44) might have expanded his statement to include all nurses when he wrote that "an aggressive attitude aimed at capturing for nursing anything that physicians might be willing to yield sole dominion over enhances nursing as a profession and the economic opportunity for nurse practitioners."

Primary Activities of Nurses in Advanced Practice

The primary activities of nurse practitioners include screening, physical and psychosocial assessment, follow-up when deviations from normal are detected, continuity of care, health promotion, problem-centered services related to diagnosis, identification, and mobilization of resources, health education, and client and group advocacy. Nurse practitioners may be involved with aspects of primary, secondary, and tertiary care (45, 46, 47, 48). Functions identified in the longitudinal study of nurse practitioners include taking a health history, performing a physical examination, patient care management, surveillance of well persons, and illness care (49). Archer and Fleshman also found nurse practitioners who were responsible for teaching other health workers and students, management of personnel and/or resources, consultation, evaluation, research planning, and administration (45, 46). In a national survey of nurse practitioners (N=5,964), Towers (50) reported that nurse practitioners "manage pharmacologic therapeutics in all fifty states, across all specialties, and in all locales..."

The role of the clinical nurse specialist encompasses a number of direct and indirect care aspects. In one review of role expectations, the authors found the clinician or direct care role to be foremost (51), with indirect role activities including consultation, staff advocacy, peer education, change agent, policy analyst, patient education, product evaluation, research, supervision, and mentoring (52, 53, 54, 55, 56, 57). Another analysis of the role activities corroborates these findings and adds the category of professional development which includes self-directed learning activities, continuing education, and writing for publication other than that associated with research (58). All of these functions relate to the scope of practice statements that have been generated by various professional organizations in attempts to provide guidelines on what it is that nurses in advanced practice roles do for their clients that is unique and different.

Scope of Practice

Scope of practice statements are based on what is legally allowable in each state under its nurse practice act. They do, however, go beyond the law in some states, as they are prepared by national professional organizations. Their intention is to provide guidelines for the practice of nursing under special conditions and with advanced preparation. These statements also may be interpreted as indicators of the expectations employers and clients may have of those who call themselves nurse practitioners or clinical nurse specialists, indicating a particular target population. In reviewing scope of practice statements, however, it is important to recognize that they are guidelines rather than mandates. Fagin (59) has written, "...nursing's scope of practice must be viewed as fluid and evolutionary."

In the 1970s, as the advanced practice movement gained momentum and programs proliferated, a number of the professional organizations, both nursing and medical, set about the task of developing scope of practice statements and guidelines for educational preparation, in particular for nurse practitioners. The American Nurses Association took the lead in developing program guidelines and scope of practice statements for college health, geriatric, adult and family, and pediatric nurse practitioners. A list of such publications is included in Appendix A. Each of these guidelines and statements addresses practice activities and settings. Concurrently, scope of practice statements were developed for specialty advanced practice. The documents may also include statements about professional responsibility, interprofessional relationships, and client advocacy. Various divisions on practice of ANA have prepared the scope documents. The one on college health is co-authored by the American College Health Association. The guidelines for educational programs address issues such as goals, planning, services and facilities, faculty, course content, admission of students, length, and evaluation.

The National Association of Pediatric Nurse Associates and Practitioners and the American Academy of Pediatrics in 1975 issued a joint statement on the scope of practice, functions, and responsibilities of pediatric nurse associates and practitioners. In 1974, ANA issued a scope of practice statement for pediatric nurse practitioners, updating it in 1980.

The Nurses' Association of the American College of Obstetricians and Gynecologists, or NAACOG (as of 1993 its name is the Association of Women's Health, Obstetric, and Neonatal Nurses; its acronym AWHONN), has taken an active role in defining practices for women's health and maternal and newborn care. In 1979, in collaboration with the American Academy of Family Physicians, the American Academy of Pediatrics, the American College of Obstetricians and Gynecologists, and NAPNAP, NAACOG issued a statement on the role definition, description, and educational guidelines for obstetric-gynecologic nurse practitioners, updating the document in 1984 and 1990. NAACOG also issued statements on the expanded role of health professionals in obstetric and gynecologic care (1980), definitions of nursing titles (including nurse practitioners), and a definition of primary health care (1979).

The American College of Nurse-Midwives administers national certification examinations, issues scope of practice statements for nurse-midwifery practice, and sets standards for educational programs, which exist both as certificate granting entities and as part of master's degree preparation.

The American Academy of Pediatrics has issued several policy statements on the practice of nurses. These include a policy on the pediatric nurse associate, a definition of pediatric nurse practitioners/associates, and a statement on the use of school nurse practitioners (see Appendix A).

Many of the more than 25 organizations that certify nurses also have prepared scope of practice statements, in addition to those cited here. Some, of course, do not specify advanced practice with educational preparation in a certificate or graduate program (60).

In 1980, the American Nurses Association Congress for Nursing Practice's scope of nursing policy statement was issued. According to this statement, "nursing is the diagnosis and treatment of human responses to actual or potential health problems" (62). This policy statement addressed the issue of specialists within nursing and recognized those nurses prepared at the graduate level and/or those certified by ANA. This document is currently being revised.

The nurse preparing for or practicing in an advanced practice role must be familiar with those scope of practice documents pertinent to her/his area of expertise. In addition to the state nurse practice acts, scope of practice statements delineate expectations, roles, and responsibilities which may reasonably be part of the practice of such a practitioner. They may provide the basis for preparing a job description, for materials to educate the public about what a nurse practitioner does, and as the basis for evaluation of practice.

It is interesting to note the intrusion of physicians and physician organizations into the arena and their attempts to define and delineate what nurses may do. Examples include statements by AAP and ACOG on the roles and scope of practice for nurse practitioners and nurse associates. We as nurses must be assertive in controlling our practice and defining what constitutes nursing. If we abdicate these responsibilities, others will take over. The efforts of the American Nurses Association and its constituent practice divisions are important to the nursing profession as a whole. Supporting the Council on Advanced Nursing Practice and/or other specialty groups for advanced practice is one way to assure that nurses retain control over nursing.

Interdisciplinary Aspects of the Role

Since the formal conceptualization of the advanced practice roles in 1954 and 1965, collaboration has been an integral part of those roles. It is inherent in the definition of primary care. According to the definition prepared by the ANA Congress for Nursing Practice, one component of the role is "interprofessional consultation" (60). A study of clinical nurse specialists in collaborative practice illustrates the role expectations and acceptance (62). In Sultz et al.'s longitudinal study of nurse practitioners, only five percent of respondents reported that their records are never reviewed by other providers (63). By implication then, the other 95 percent have input, at least through record review, for their interactions with clients.

Mauksch has stated that the nurse/physician dyad is most important to client care. Whereas she views physicians as focusing on illness, diagnosis, treatment, and curing, nurses focus on wellness, assessment and interventions, caring, comforting, teaching, counseling, and coordinating. She went on to state that physicians must move to viewing nurses as colleagues, to saying "we" rather than "I," from "what's in it for me" to "what is best for the client," and to learn respect for clients as human beings (64). Mauksch points out that physicians are not always interested in collaboration, however, and may even actively oppose nurse practitioners (65).

One of the reasons that interdisciplinary collaboration is so important to the roles in advanced practice is the responsibility for continuity and coordination of care inherent in providing primary care or in case management. It becomes a critical issue for nurses serving as primary care providers or case managers because overlap of functions is more obvious in these roles than for nurses in other areas. Additionally, nurses now are prepared to assume responsibility for components of care that were previously the sole domain of physicians, such as physical examinations. Conflicts over territoriality are common as health care providers are reluctant to yield turf or recognize the expertise of others (66). As Challela (67) noted, nurses have often relied on being liked rather than on being evaluated objectively for the contributions they make to client care based on expertise and knowledge.

In 1972, the National Joint Practice Commission first met, with eight representatives from nursing and eight from medicine, under sponsorship and funding from the ANA and AMA. Activities over the 10-year existence of the commission included joint practice conferences, publication of a casebook on joint practice, and a project to demonstrate collaboration in hospital settings. In 1980, the AMA voted to withdraw financial support and in February 1981 support ended (68).

The now defunct National Joint Practice Commission defined joint practice as "nurses and physicians collaborating as colleagues to provide patient care" (69). To adopt the view that nurses, physicians, or any one type of professional health care provider can provide for all of the health care needs of an individual, family, group, or community over an extended period of time is exceedingly myopic. Thus, nurses in advanced practice roles have been forced, by the very nature of their practice as case managers, to seek collaborative working relationships with other providers, particularly physicians.

A variety of associations is possible. Nurses may establish joint practices with other providers. They may utilize, and in turn be utilized by, others as consultants. Nurse practitioners and clinical nurse specialists may be employed by physicians, clinics, health maintenance organizations, nursing homes, or other institutions not controlled by nurses, or may contract with agencies or institutions to obtain certain services for their clients or to deliver certain services. It is possible for nurses to form partnerships or corporations (70). Relationships may also be much less formal, as when all providers are employees of an agency or institution such as a neighborhood health center, clinic, or health maintenance organization.

Joint practice between nurses and physicians has received much attention in the literature. Since "nursing and medicine have the longest traditions and the greatest numbers," it is not surprising that attention is focused on the relationship between these two groups of professionals (71). The nurse practitioner role as it evolved in the 1960s grew out of a collaborative effort between physicians and a nurse faculty person interested in the care of children in the community. Many of the early programs utilized and even required physician preceptors since there were, of course, few nurse preceptors available at first. Because clinical nurse specialists evolved out of advanced practice and specialty roles in secondary and tertiary settings, preceptorships were often less troublesome to find among nurses. An exception might be psychiatric-mental health nursing with blurring of roles as primary therapist with the psychiatrist, psychologist, and psychiatric social worker (72).

It is important to recognize and acknowledge that, in a sense, the roles of physician and nurse *are* competitive. Nurses are and will be competing for office space, organizational support, a share of the health care dollar, and a voice in decision making for health policies at all levels. Nurses and physicians must, however, be collaborative and collegial as well as competitive if goals for client care are to be accomplished (73).

When the National Joint Practice Commission began to study joint practice in 1973, efforts were made to identify such practices in order to collect data. Over 250 nurse/ physician practices were identified (74). Selected cases from the study are published in *Together* (74). They illustrate how physicians and nurses can collaborate as colleagues with the common goal of giving sensitive, high quality care for clients in a variety of settings, from suburbia to the mountains of Tennessee, utilizing a number of models for the relationships, ranging from teams to a single nurse/physician duo.

Steel (75) describes the developmental stages for joint practice: negotiation of the contract, contract implementation, and refinement. Steel points out that it is important for health care professionals considering joint practice to recognize the need for each of these steps to occur, to plan for them, and to evaluate both process and content of the arrangement on an ongoing basis. Steel points out that a basic level of understanding and trust and respect for territory are necessary for a joint practice to succeed.

Collaborative relationships with other members of the health care team are inherent in and essential to the role of nurses in advanced practice. Whether these are intra- or interdisciplinary, such relationships are implied in the delivery of primary care and in case management models. Interpretation of the role of the nurse to other providers constitutes an important component of the collaborative process.

The ANA publication, *Nursing: A Social Policy Statement* (1980), defines collaboration as "true partnership," one in which both sides have and value power, recognize and accept separate and combined spheres of responsibility and activity, safeguard mutually the interests of each, and share common goals. Such a relationship thrives on the richness each lends to the other because of the strengths and uniqueness each can contribute to the whole (76). One of the goals for advanced practice nurses in role development is establishing such relationships with physicians and other providers.

Acceptance of Nurse Practitioners and Clinical Nurse Specialists by Other Providers

Nurse practitioners and clinical nurse specialists experience varying degrees of acceptance of their new role by other providers. A number of surveys and studies have been conducted which looked at the acceptance of such nurses by others, in particular by physicians. Simmons and Rosenthal (77) found that nurse practitioners whom they interviewed perceived trust on the part of some physicians and total rejection by others. Those who perceived distrust characterized their working relationships with physicians as good, but hastened to add that they work with a biased sample.

The acceptance of pediatric nurse practitioners by pediatricians was explored in a study conducted by Claiborn and Walton (78). They found that physicians in nonprivate practice and subspecialty practice and those working with poverty level clients were more accepting, as were those who were younger and had been in practice a short time. The physicians who were rated as antipractitioner felt the concept would alter physician-client relationships and that quality would be sacrificed for quantity.

In another study (79), the physicians surveyed were found to hold generally positive attitudes toward nurse practitioners. Most of them indicated a preference for nurse practitioners in an employee role. Some reluctance to give up authority and to see the nurse as an independent professional with different but important contributions to make was evident.

A longitudinal study on nurse practitioners (80) produced some interesting results. Employers overwhelmingly (93%) reported that the benefits of having nurse practitioners outweighed the costs. Interestingly, employers were more likely than the nurse practitioners themselves to believe that the role was accepted by physicians and members of the community. Both employers and nurse practitioners believed clients to be the most accepting group.

Nurse practitioners and their employers agreed that resistance from other health providers constitutes one barrier to role development (81). Similarly, clinical nurse specialists identified rejection by other providers as an impediment to integration into the system and role implementation in general (82, 83).

Acceptance of nurse practitioners and clinical nurse specialists by associates is evident in data collected through the Yale experience in educating nurses for new roles. Measures of acceptance included referrals from other providers, ratings as to contribution to overall patient care, contribution to day-to-day operations in outpatient clinics, and task delegation (84).

One component of a study of clinical nurse specialists in collaborative practice was physician acceptance. The authors found physicians to be satisfied. The clinical nurse specialists in the sample felt physicians' expectations were appropriate (85).

Relationships between these nurses and other providers, particularly physicians, can be characterized in a number of ways. Little (86) has categorized them as: guest, colleague, gatekeeper, and manager. Whereas all relationships may have some of each of these components, role development will be influenced by the degree to which each is present or dominant over the others. Those nurses who are primarily guests in a physician's private practice will find themselves constrained in role development. Control is not shared but remains primarily with the physician. Rules are established by the host (86).

The nurse may serve in a gatekeeper role for an agency, or that position may be relegated to another provider. These settings tend to be highly formalized and have many structural controls built into the system (86). Often the consistent providers are the nurses whose investment is greater than that of the transients in the system. Role development may then be constrained by the system. On the other hand, if nurses have longevity as providers, they may use the advantage of accrued seniority and familiarity to establish the rules, develop protocols, and control their own practice in a collegial relationship with physicians (85).

The nurse whose role includes management activities may also find that she or he represents stability within the provider population. A survey of clinical nurse specialists three to five years after graduation demonstrated roles in administration, especially in planning and policy making (87). Advantages may result from continuity of contact with clients and investment in the position over time. Role development and acceptance by other providers as colleagues may result from the nurse's position as a manager and the relative power within the system. Skillful assertiveness combined with success in the managerial aspects of the role can result in respect from other providers (86).

Awareness of the possible patterns of relationships will enable the advanced practice nurse to assess the potential for role development and acceptance by other providers of that role during job interviews. To some degree, patterns can be predicted if one makes inquiries about organizational structure and process, case-load assignment, consultation, economic terms, and the philosophy of care. Exploring the controls which regulate the access of each provider to clients will help the nurse evaluate how the nurse's advanced role will be accepted by those with whom she or he will be working most closely and what potential there will be for change (85, 86).

Socialization into the Role. Assuming roles that are only a few decades old and which are still a source of confusion for both the public and other providers is an awesome prospect. The need for nurse practitioner and clinical nurse specialist students to explore those components of the role beyond the hands-on client care is evident in their obsession with questions such as, How do I define my role to others? What do I do if I am expected to perform activities for which I have not been prepared? Identifying generic professional behaviors can be helpful in analyzing advanced practice roles (88).

One of the problems in preparing nurses as advanced practice specialists and socializing them into the role is the paucity of faculty with active practices who can act as role models for collegiality in practice with other providers, especially physicians (89). In 1977, the Robert Wood Johnson Foundation initiated funding for a year-long fellowship program to prepare faculty in primary care. These fellowships afforded faculty the opportunity to prepare for and practice the role of primary care provider in a collaborative relationship (90). By increasing the emphasis on clinical practice and reward systems for faculty who maintain an active practice, the availability of models can be increased. Innovative approaches to faculty practice through joint appointments (91), shared practices with other providers, demonstration interdisciplinary teams, and the creation of nursing wellness centers and other nurse-managed practice models all provide means for faculty to carry a practice and retain clinical competence. The availability of faculty role models enhances the educational process and socializes students into all aspects of the role of nurse practitioner or clinical nurse specialist, clinical and nonclinical.

Students in graduate programs need opportunities to explore the nonclinical aspects of their roles. After the initial focus on client assessment and management skills, students need to move on to role construction (92). At the same time, it is important to recognize that the nurse in advanced practice must ultimately define his or her role and realize that the role is "a negotiative process undertaken in the context of an actual work situation" (93).

Part of socialization involves the opportunity for role practice and role negotiation. These experiences can be built into an educational program. The art of negotiation is useful at all levels of practice, from one-on-one relationships to the macro system level and can be taught in graduate programs (94). Opportunities to apply one's knowledge in as realistic a setting as possible are critical to learning about one's role (95, 96).

Some of the role-related issues which have been identified during the process of role acquisition include increased responsibility for client care inherent in providing primary care or serving as a case manager;

changing relationships with other providers, particularly physicians; alterations in relationships with significant others (96); public concepts of what a nurse practitioner or clinical nurse specialist is and does; and how to negotiate the role without detriment to employment opportunities. Discussion about role definition and negotiation should be part of the educational process for becoming an advanced practice nurse (96, 97). Such discussion might also be an integral part of continuing education programs for nurse practitioners and clinical nurse specialists. Indeed, we should not forget the needs of nurses already in advanced practice roles for preparation for and opportunity for role advancement (98). Faculty might even facilitate mentor relationships for students (see Chapter 11).

Summary

The content and process of role implementation are important issues for the individual practicing in an advanced role. "Nursing is not second-class medicine, but first-class health care" (99). Ford has pointed out that the role of the nurse in advanced practice is not well understood and that nurses themselves are not always clear about their roles and are, therefore, allowing the system to use them inappropriately (100).

Role conflicts and role negotiations are a way of life for these nurses. We can expect to expend considerable energy trying to get physicians, other providers, and the public to understand who we are and what we have to offer. Those of us who serve as role models, as faculty and preceptors, must help prepare our students for the problems inherent in role change. Support for and interpretation of new roles is, at least in part, the responsibility of nursing leadership (101). Nurses in advanced practice have a great deal to offer to the public in expertise and wellness and illness care. We are the ones responsible for delineating and defining our roles and scope of practice, for determining settings, and for educating other providers and the general public.

REFERENCES

1. Ford, L.C. (1979). A nurse for all settings: The nurse practitioner. Nursing Outlook 27:516-521.

2. Brown, E.L. (1949). Nursing for the Future. New York: Russell Sage. p. 100.
3. Breckinridge, M. (1952). Wide Neighborhoods. New York: Harper and Brothers.
4. Ford, L.C. & Silver, H.K. (1967). Expanded role of the nurse in child care. Nursing Outlook 15:43-45.
5. Mayo, A.A. (1944). Advanced courses in clinic nursing. American Journal of Nursing 44(6):579-585.
6. Beecroft, P.C. & Papenhausen, J.L. (1989). Who is a clinical nurse specialist? Clinical Nurse Specialist 4(3):103-104.
7. Montemuro, M.A. (1987). The evolution of the clinical nurse specialist: Response to the challenge of professional nursing practice. Clinical Nurse Specialist 1(3):106-110.
8. Martin, E.J. (1985). "A specialty in decline?" Journal of Professional Nursing 9(1):48-53.
9. Levine, E. (1977). What do we know about nurse practitioners? American Journal of Nursing 77:1799-1803.
10. Walker, A.E. (1972). PRIMEX - the family nurse practitioner program. Nursing Outlook 20:28-31.
11. Preparing nurses for family health care. (1972). Nursing Outlook 20:53-56.
12. American Nurses' Association Congress for Nursing Practice (1974). Definition: Nurse practitioner, nurse clinician and clinical nurse specialist. Kansas City, MO: American Nurses' Association.
13. Jones, F.M. (1981). ANA's certification for specialization. In: J.C. McCloskey & H.K. Grace (Eds.), Current Issues in Nursing. Boston: Blackwell Scientific. pp. 353-359.
14. Allen, E.A. (1977). Credentialing of continuing education nurse practitioner programs. In: A.A. Bliss and E.D. Cohen (Eds.), The New Health Professionals. Germantown, MD: Aspen. p. 83.
15. Safriet, B.J. (1992). Health care dollars and regulatory sense. Yale Journal on Regulation 9:417-488.
16. American Nurses' Association and U.S. Department of Health, Education and Welfare. (1974). A Directory of Programs Preparing Registered Nurses for Expanded Roles, 1973-1974. Bethesda, MD: U.S. Department of Health, Education and Welfare.
17. Golden, A.S. (1979). The impact of new health professionals. In:

Health Care in the 1980s. Who Provides? Who Plans? Who Pays? New York: National League for Nursing. pp. 46-47.
18. National League for Nursing (1992). Nursing Data Review 1992. New York: NLN.
19. American Nurses Association (1989). Directory of Accredited Organizations and Continuing Education Certificate Programs Preparing Nurse Practitioners. Kansas City, MO: ANA.
20. Forbes, K.E., Rafson, J., Spross, J.A. & Kozlowski, D. (1990). Clinical nurse specialist and nurse practitioner core curricula survey results. The Nurse Practitioner 15(4):43;46-48.
21. National League for Nursing position statement on the education of nurse practitioners. (1979). New York: National League for Nursing.
22. Pearson, L.J. (1993). 1992-93 update: How each state stands on legislative issues affecting advanced nursing practice. The Nurse Practitioner 18(1):23-28;30-32;35-36;38.
23. American Nurses Association (1989). Directory of Accredited Organizations and Continuing Education Certificate Programs Preparing Nurse Practitioners. Kansas City, MO; ANA.
24. National League for Nursing (1992, See ref. 18).
25. American Nurses Association (1989, see ref. 19).
26. Sultz, H.A., Henry, O.M., Kinyon, L.J., Buck, G.M. & Bullough, B. (1983). A decade of change for nurse practitioners. Nursing Outlook 31(3):137-141.
27. Sparacino, P. & Durand, B.A. (1986). Specialization in advanced practice. CPHCNP Newsletter 9:(2):3-4.
28. Hawkins, J.E. & Rafson, J. (1991). ANA council merger creates council of nurses in advanced practice. Clinical Nurse Specialist 5(3):131-132.
29. Rafson, J. (1990). NP/CNS Council merger. CPHCNP Newsletter 13(2):1;6.
30. Hanson, C. & Martin, L.L. (1990). The nurse practitioner and clinical nurse specialist: Should the roles be merged? Journal of the American Academy of Nurse Practitioners 2(1):2-9.
31. Elder, R.G. & Bullough, B. (1990). Nurse practitioners and clinical nurse specialists: Are the role merging? Clinical Nurse Specialist 4(2):78-84.
32. Diers, D. (1985). Preparation of practitioners, clinical specialists,

and clinicians. Journal of Professional Nursing 1(1):41.
33. Diers, 1985, op cit, p. 47.
34. Kinlein, M.L. (1972). Independent nurse practitioner. Nursing Outlook 20:22-24.
35. Alford, D.M. & Jensen, M.J. (1976). Reflections on private practice. American Journal of Nursing 76:1966-1968.
36. Jacox, A.K. & Norris, C.M. (Eds.) (1977). Organizing for Independent Nursing Practice. New York: Appleton-Century-Crofts. pp. 2-6.
37. Facts about Nursing 86-87. (1987). Kansas City, MO: American Nurses' Association.
38. Hodnicki, D. (1988). Nurses - meeting the needs of the homeless. Newsletter of the Council of Primary Health Care Nurse Practitioners 11(3):1.
39. Durham, J.D. & Hardin, S.B. (1985). Promoting advanced nursing practice. The Nurse Practitioner 10(12):59-62.
40. Hagan, P.C. (1989). The growth of clinical nurse specialist interest groups. Momentum 6(2):1-2.
41. Rew, L. (1988). AFFIRM the role of clinical specialist in private practice. Clinical Nurse Specialist 2(1):39-43.
42. Ball, G.B. (1990). Perspectives on developing, marketing, and implementing a new clinical nurse specialist position. Clinical Nurse Specialist 4(1):33-36.
43. Towers, J. (1990). Report of the national survey of the American Academy of Nurse Practitioners, Part IV: Practice characteristics and marketing activities of nurse practitioners. Journal of the American Academy of Nurse Practitioners 2(4):164-167.
44. Hershey, N (1980). A health lawyer's view. Nursing Law and Ethics 1:1,5.
45. Archer, S.E. & Fleshman R.P. (1975). Community health nursing: A typology of practice. Nursing Outlook 23:358-364.
46. Archer, S.E. (1976). Community nurse practitioner: Another assessment. Nursing Outlook 24:499-503.
47. Levine, J.I., Orr, S.T. Sheatsley, D.W., Lohr, J.A. & Brodie, B.M. (1978). The nurse practitioner: Role, physician utilization, patient acceptance. Nursing Research 27:245-254.
48. Southby, J.R. (1980). Primary care nurse practitioners within the Army health care system: Expectations and perceptions of role.

Military Medicine 145:659-665.
49. Sultz, H.A., Zielezny, M., Gentry, J.M. & Kinyon, L. (1980). Longitudinal Study of Nurse Practitioners (Phase III). Hyattsville, MD: U.S. Department of Health, Education and Welfare. pp. 29-30.
50. Towers, J. (1991). Report of the national survey of the American Academy of Nurse Practitioners, Part II: Pharmacologic management practices. Journal of the American Academy of Nurse Practitioners 1(4):137.
51. Burge, S., Crigler, L., Hurt, L., Kelly, G. & Sanborn, C. (1989). Clinical nurse specialist role development: Quantifying actual practice over three years. Clinical Nurse Specialist 3(1):33-36.
52. Topham, D.L. (1987). Role theory in relation to roles of the clinical nurse specialist. Clinical Nurse Specialist 1(2):81-84.
53. Beyerman, K.L. (1988). Consultation roles of the clinical nurse specialist: A case study. Clinical Nurse Specialist 2(2):91-95.
54. Brandt, P.A. & Magyard, D.L. (1989). Preparation of clinical nurse specialists for family-centered early intervention. Infants and Young Children 1(3):51-62.
55. Stimpson, M. & Hanley, B. (1991). Nurse policy analyst: Advanced practice role. Nursing & Health Care 12(1):10-15.
56. Harrison, E.A. (1989). Product evaluation and the clinical nurse specialists: An opportunity for role development. Clinical Nurse Specialist 3(2):85-89.
57. Storr, G. (1988). The clinical nurse specialists: From the outside looking up. Journal of Advanced Nursing 13:265-272.
58. Robichaud, A. & Hamric, A.B. (1986). Time documentation of clinical nurse specialist activities. Journal of Nursing Administration 16(1):31-36.
59. Fagin, C.M. (1977). Nature and scope of nursing practice in meeting primary health care needs. In: Primary Care by Nurses: Sphere of Responsibility and Accountability. Kansas City, MO: American Academy of Nursing. p. 39.
60. Nursing: A social policy statement. (1980). Kansas City, MO: American Nurses' Association.
61. Styles, M.M. (1989). On Specialization in Nursing: Toward a New Empowerment. Kansas City, MO: American Nurses' Foundation.
62. Riegel, B. & Murrell, T. (1987). Clinical nurse specialists in

collaborative practice. Clinical Nurse Specialist 1(2):63-69.
63. Sultz, H.A., Zielezny, M., Gentry, J.M. & Kinyon, L. (1980). (see ref. 49), p. 31.
64. Mauksch, I.G. (1977). Unpublished speech given at Alpha Chi Chapter, Sigma Theta Tau, Boston College, MA., Feb. 28.
65. Mauksch, I.G. (1978). The nurse practitioner movement - where does it go from here? American Journal of Public Health 68:1074-1075.
66. Gardner, H.H. & Fiske, M.S. (1981). Pluralism and competition: A possibility for primary care. American Journal of Nursing 81:2152-2157.
67. Challela, M. (1979). The interdisciplinary team: A role definition for nursing. Image 11:9-15.
68. National League for Nursing position statement on the education of nurse practitioners. (1979). New York: National League for Nursing.
69. Melvin, N. (1979). Developing guidelines for clinical privileges for nurse practitioners. In: Power: Nursing's Challenge for Change. Kansas City, MO: American Nurses' Association. p. 66.
70. Jacox, K. & Norris, C.M. op. cit. (see Ref. 36), pp. 75-104.
71. Bates, B. (1972). Nurse-physician dyad: Collegial or competitive? In: Three Challenges to the Nursing Profession. New York: American Nurses' Association. p. 5.
72. Martin (1985, see ref. 8).
73. Bates (1972. see ref. 71).
74. Roueche, B. (Ed.) (1977). Together: A Casebook of Joint Practices in Primary Care. Chicago: The National Practice Commission. pp. vii, 2-16.
75. Steel, J.E. (1981). Putting joint practice into practice. American Journal of Nursing 81:964-967.
76. American Nurses' Association Congress for Nursing Practice (1980, see Ref. 60).
77. Simmons, R.S. & Rosenthal, J. (1981). The women's movement and the nurse practitioner's sense of role. Nursing Outlook 29:371-375.
78. Claiborn, S.A. & Walton, W. (1979). Pediatrician's acceptance of PNPs. American Journal of Nursing 79:300.
79. Sides, D.A. (1980). Attitudes of Portland area physicians toward

nurses in expanded roles. Western Journal of Nursing Research 2:730-737.
80. Sultz, H.A., Zielezny, M., Gentry, J.M. & Kinyon, L. (1980). op. cit. (see Ref. 49), p. 32.
81. Ibid., p. 33.
82. Page, N.E. & Arena, D.M. (1991). Practical strategies for CNS role implementation. Clinical Nurse Specialist 5(1):43-48.
83. Harrell, J.S. & McCulloch, S.D. (1986). The role of the clinical nurse specialist: Problems and solutions. Journal of Nursing Administration 16(10:44-48.
84. Storms, D.M. (1973). Training of the Nurse Practitioner: A Clinical and Statistical Analysis. New Haven, CT: Health Services Research. pp. 77-96.
85. Riegel, B. & Murrell, T. (1987). op. cit. (see ref. 62), p. 67.
86. Little, M. (1980). Nurse practitioner/physician relationships. American Journal of Nursing 80:1642-1645.
87. Radke, K., McArt, E., Schmitt, M. & Walker, E.K. (1990). Administrative preparation of clinical nurse specialists. Journal of Professional Nursing 6(4):221-228.
88. O'Rourke, M.W. (1989). Generic professional behaviors: Implications for the clinical nurse specialist role. Clinical Nurse Specialist 3(3):128-132.
89. Ford, L.C. (1979, see ref. 1).
90. Keenan, T. (1978). Birth of the fellowship program. In: Nurse Faculty Fellowships in Primary Care. Robert Wood Johnson Foundation, First Annual Symposium. pp. 22-23.
91. Minarik, P.A. (1990). Collaboration between service and education: Perils or pleasures for the clinical nurse specialist? Clinical Nurse Specialist 4(2):109-114.
92. Ryan-Merritt, M.V., Mitchell, C.A. & Pagel, I. (1988). Clinical nurse specialist role definition and operationalization. Clinical Nurse Specialist 2(3):132-138.
93. Knafl, K.A. (1978). How nurse practitioner students construct their role. Nursing Outlook 26:650-653.
94. Beare, P.G. (1989). The essentials of the win-win negotiation for the clinical nurse specialist. Clinical Nurse Specialist 3(3):138-141.
95. Knafl, K.A. (1979). How real is the practicum for nurse practitioner students? Nursing Outlook 27:131-135.

96. Ryan-Merritt, M.V., Mitchell, C.A. & Pagel, I. (1988)(See Ref. 92).
97. Lukacs, J.L. (1982). Factors in nurse practitioner role adjustment. The Nurse Practitioner 7:2-23, 50.
98. Oda, D.S., Sparacino, P.S.A. & Boyd, P. (1988). Role advancement for the experienced clinical nurse specialist. Clinical Nurse Specialist 2:167-171.
99. Ford, L.C. (Nov. 13, 1980). Wellness: A focus for nursing practice. Unpublished paper presented at Wellness:Focus for the 80s. American Nurses' Association Annual Conference for the Council of Primary Health Care Nurse Practitioners. Philadelphia.
100. An interview with Dr. Loretta Ford. (1975). The Nurse Practitioner 1:9-12.
101. Moore, A.C. (1974). Nurse practitioner: Reflections on the role. Nursing Outlook 22:124-127.

BIBLIOGRAPHY

Competencies and Program Guidelines for Nurse Providers of Childbirth Education. (1987). Washington, DC: NAACOG.

Goertzen, I.E. (1991). Differentiating Nursing Practice into the Twenty-First Century. Kansas City, MO: American Academy of Nursing.

Hamric, A.B. & Spross, J.A. (Eds.) (1989). The Clinical Nurse Specialist in Theory and Practice. 2nd ed. Philadelphia: Saunders.

Hardy, M.E. & Conway, M.E. (1988). Role Theory: Perspectives for the Health Professionals. 2nd ed. Norwalk, CT: Appleton & Lange.

Menard, S.W. (1987). The Clinical Nurse Specialist. Perspectives on Practice. New York: Wiley.

Nurse Providers of Neonatal Care. Guidelines for Educational Development and Practice. (1990). Washington, DC: NAACOG.

The Obstetric-Gynecologic Women's Health Nurse Practitioner. (1990). Washington, DC: NAACOG.

Practice Competencies and Educational Guidelines for Nurse Providers of Intrapartum care. (1987). Washington, DC: NAACOG.

The Role of the Clinical Nurse Specialist. (1986). Kansas City, MO:

3

Effects of Sex-Role Stereotyping on Leadership in Nursing: Need for a Feminist Paradigm *[1]

Introduction

In this chapter we will discuss the pervasive and persistent nature of sex discrimination which has affected the nursing profession's ability to influence issues relating to health care delivery. A major issue is the advanced practitioner's autonomy vis-a-vis a male dominated medical profession. Knowledge about sex-role stereotyping and the effects it has on leadership in nursing can assist the practitioner and clinical specialist to develop strategies for gaining influence in health care settings.

Sex-Role Stereotyping: Women and Nursing

Ninety-seven percent of nurses are women (1). As recently as 1972,

---

* With Pauline F. Hebert, Ph.D.

[1] In this chapter the practitioner or clinical specialist is referred to as "she" because the chapter deals with women and sex-role stereotyping. There is no intent to disregard the male nurse.

research studies revealed that "existing stereotypic differences between men and women are approved of and even idealized by large segments of our society" (2). Sex-role stereotypes not only affect the way people perceive the behavior of others as being appropriate or inappropriate but they also influence whether they classify such behavior as healthy or unhealthy.

Sex-role stereotypes are dangerous cultural social patterns not only because they limit opportunities but also because they affect achievement and motivation and ultimately affect the self-esteem of otherwise healthy and competent women. Proponents of the ERA (Equal Rights Amendment) are still struggling to achieve a legislative mandate to guarantee equal opportunity for women, but it is doubtful whether a law alone can reverse the tide and put to rest the myths supporting the contention that women are biologically and intellectually inferior to men.

In nursing, women have played games with physicians, allowing themselves to assume and maintain positions of subservience which foster attitudes of medical paternalism in their professional relationships. Such behaviors may have been appropriate for survival in past centuries but the needs and issues which will have to be addressed in the health care setting of the twenty-first century require a change in functional role and subsequent changes in interpersonal relationships.

Women continue to be perceived as less competent, less independent, less objective and less logical then men (2). One of the major difficulties which exists today is the unavailability of an appropriate tool to fairly evaluate women. "Women are studied—and study themselves—in terms of masculine constructs" (3). These tools have been shown to incorporate masculine bias so that "...female can only come out as 'not male'" (3). Broverman states that:

> Women are clearly put in a double bind by the fact that different standards exist for women than for adults. If women adopt the behaviors specified as desirable for adults, they risk censure for their failure to be appropriately feminine, but if they adopt the behaviors that are designated as feminine, they are necessarily deficient with respect to the general standards for adult behavior (4).

Virginia Cleland (5) classifies sex discrimination as nursing's most pervasive problem and states that nursing's autonomy is a false premise since the important decisions for nurses and nursing are not made by its members. The nursing profession and its members have assumed, more often than not, a reactive position, allowing more powerful groups the privileges of decision-making and offensive action. In a recent successful suit filed against a Connecticut hospital on the grounds of negligence by an employed nurse, a hospital regulation was subsequently adopted requiring a *physician* to double check medications prescribed prior to administration (6). In October 1977, although two nurse practitioners were functioning legally within the framework of the New Jersey state nurse practice act in an HMO setting, the Board of State Medical Examiners nevertheless filed charges against both of them, accusing each of practicing medicine without a license (7). Both of these examples portray the defensive positions nurses so often find themselves in.

For too long, physicians have assumed the right to dictate nursing's role. When something unfortunate happens, as in the Connecticut hospital situation described above, they quickly take action to keep nursing professionals under the thumb of medicine. What little autonomy has been demonstrated in nursing has been allowed by physicians as a means of meeting their own needs and goals. Although recent changes in most state nurse practice acts have acknowledged independent functions for nursing, physicians continue to challenge these. Analyzing this situation, Edmonds (8) draws the conclusion that physicians perceive nurse practitioner and clinical specialist functions as behaviors which indirectly impinge upon their power. She compares patients to resources and nurse access to patients as threats to the medical ownership of patients.

It seems reasonable to argue that a predominantly male medical profession is at odds with a predominantly female nursing profession for reasons which transcend professional interests and needs and are deeply rooted in sexual discrimination. Ashley even claims that this is more than it appears to be and represents, in addition, misogyny (9).

Women and Society

Depressed women outnumber men by two to one (10). In a study of women physicians and Ph.D.s, 51% of women physicians and 32% of women Ph.D.s were significantly depressed and related their depression to sex discrimination in their work setting (11). In another study, female physicians had a suicide rate 6.56% higher than male physicians and four time higher than American women in the same age range (12). It seems evident that sex discrimination affects even the most highly educated and competent women in American society, damaging their self-esteem and emotional and mental health.

Women and Other Women

That successful women encounter prejudice and discrimination from males is a difficult enough situation. It is often true, however, that females tend to judge successful women just as harshly. There is no "old boy" network of women to latch onto for encouragement and support. LeRoux (1) discusses the way women are prejudiced against other women, undermining themselves and others by using censure whenever a woman violates a stereotype. Sohier (13) is concerned with how nurses can imbue each other with shared power and a community based on trust. The legacy of patriarchal rule is nurses' distrust of other nurses. "Revaluing" other nurses and becoming increasingly aware of the power inherent in our different perspectives can sustain change to a supporting, caring, trusting community and empower nurses to change the face of health care.

Women and Economics

According to statistics, nursing ranks highest in prestige among the predominantly female professions, but it falls far short of the most prestigious male group, namely, physicians (14). The undervaluation of all work performed by women can easily be proven by analyzing salaries paid to males and females for performing identical tasks. Levitin, Quinn, and Stains (15) found, in an analysis of salaries for men and women, that a $4,372 mean difference existed between male and female workers; only $914 of the difference could be attributed to achievement factors while a $3,458 disparity existed for illegitimate or discriminatory reasons, leading them to conclude that most women were receiving far less income than they deserve. Without a doubt, an individual's self-esteem is closely tied to the economic worth of her or his occupational knowledge and skills. An androcentric society which places women at an economic disadvantage and where high economic rewards are far more easily attained by males is perpetuating a work environment which furthers the advantage of one group at the cost of another group.

In 1945, nurses' salaries were one-third that of physicians'. Today, nurses' economic rewards average one-fifth that of physicians' despite the fact that nurses have assumed more complex functions and are more highly educated than in years past (16). Whereas the gap between physicians' and nurses' salaries has widened, the gap between professional nurses' salaries and those of auxiliary nursing personnel has narrowed to the extent that LPNs in 1981 made 76% of professional nurses' salaries (16). By 1992, LVNs in hospitals made 63% of what RNs made (17).

In 1979, nurses' salaries were equivalent to secretaries' and significantly less than those of social workers, physical therapists, occupational therapists, and pharmacists (16). Public awareness of the worth and need for nurses has had no significant effect on society's willingness to reward nurses financially for the vital functions they perform. This economic undervaluation remains a disturbing example of sex discrimination in the work setting. A 1992 salary survey indicated significant gains: mean salaries for nurse practitioners in hospitals were $41,887 and for clinical nurse specialists, $43,593 (17). In Chapter Nine, a tool is provided for assessing a practitioner's financial worth vis-a-vis the number of clients seen and the amount of income generated by the nurse in a particular work setting. Although the nursing shortage in the 1980s led to higher entry-level salaries, the disparity in salary between experienced nurses and experts in other professions still exists.

Implications of Sex-role Stereotyping on Leadership in Nursing

The nurse practitioner or clinical specialist who attempts to exert leadership has many problems. An obvious one is the lack of available clinical nursing role models upon which to pattern a leadership style. In the past, educators, administrators, and researchers served as nursing leaders and spokespersons for the profession. This will not suffice in the future because changes in health care delivery systems will pivot around clinical issues which directly affect consumers of nursing care. Clinically oriented nurses must therefore learn to assume positions of prominence within the profession at large.

The advanced practitioner has been found to be different from her nursing peers in that she is more self-reliant, aggressive, and competitive (18). Nurse practitioners and, indeed, clinical nurse specialists, appear to be better armed to deal with issues of sexism as they attempt to gain more influence in the health care setting. While these nurses appear to possess the traits associated with leadership, their success will depend upon a variety of functions and roles which they must assume in addition to their clinical roles and everyday nursing functions.

The battle for leadership must be waged on several fronts. At the client's bedside, the nurse must articulate who she is and what her functions are. She must demonstrate excellence in practice by considering all the needs of a patient — from preventing illness, through acuity and/or chronicity of illness, and into the realms of health restoration or a peaceful and dignified death.

With physicians and other health care providers, she must be assertive in articulating her personal philosophy of nursing. She must break loose from medical paternalism and assume a more protective and assertive stance as patient advocate by leaving behind loyalties to institution and physician.

Within the profession at large, the advanced practitioner can make other nurses aware that practitioners are legitimate nurses, putting to rest the notion that they are nothing but "junior doctors." The nurse practitioner and clinical specialist need to actively participate not only at the specialty council level but also within professional organizations.

Visibility as a practitioner or clinician who can demonstrate concern and interest in issues which affect the broad scope of nursing practice is also important. It is time for the profession to pull down the walls which separate its members into isolated special interest groups. The advanced practitioner can lead the way in this endeavor (19).

The nurse practitioner or clinical specialist must extend her knowledge by increasing her awareness of societal organizations within which nurses must function. She can learn to identify where power resides in these organizations and how this power can be mobilized to further the aims of nursing. Additionally, she can work to increase her consciousness regarding subtle aspects of sex discrimination in the work setting and, when it does occur, fight against it so that nurses can achieve the success and financial rewards they deserve.

Summary

In relation to the approximately two million nurses in the United States, advanced practitioners and clinical specialists represent a very small minority. Leadership is a viable option for all practitioners and clinical specialists who possess advanced practice skills and a strong knowledge base in the fundamentals of leadership. "It is imperative that nurses recognize the value and legitimacy of their own voices. Political action by nurses requires bold actions based on visions that reflect both feminist views of the world and nursing's commitment to caring" (20).

REFERENCES

1. LeRoux, R. (1976). Sex-role stereotyping and leadership. Nursing Administration Quarterly 1:21-29.
2. Broverman, I., Vogel, S., Broverman, D., Clarkson, F., & Rosenkrantz, P. (1975). Sex-role stereotypes: A current appraisal. In: M. Mednick, S. Tangri, & L. Hoffman (Eds.), Women and Achievement. New York:Wiley and Sons. p.38.

3. Carlson, R. (1975). Understanding women: Implications for personality theory and research. In: M. Mednick, S. Tangri, & L. Hoffman (Eds.), Women and Achievement. New York:Wiley and Sons. pp. 20-21.
4. Broverman, I., Vogel, S. Broverman, D., Clarkson, F. & Rosenkrantz, P., op cit., p. 45.
5. Cleland, V. (1971). Sex discrimination: Nursing's most pervasive problem. American Journal of Nursing 71:1542-1547.
6. Demensey, G. (1981). Suit over death of a child settled. The Hartford Courant, Sept. 25, p. B1.
7. Adler, J. (1979). Guest editorial: "You are charged with..." Nurse Practitioner 4:6.
8. Edmunds, M. (1981). Non-clinical problems: Concepts of power. Nurse Practitioner 6:45-49.
9. Ashley, J. (1980). Power in structured misogyny. Implications for the politics of care. Advances in Nursing Science 2:3-22.
10. Weissman, M. & Klerman, G. (1977). Sex differences and the epidemiology of depression. Archives of General Psychiatry 34:98-111.
11. Welner, A., Martin S., Wochnik, E., Davis, M., Fishman, R. & Clayton, P. (1979). Psychiatric disorders among professional women. Archives of General Psychiatry 36:169-172.
12. Pitts, F., Schuller, B., Rich, C. & Pitts, A. (1979). Suicide among U.S. women physicians. American Journal of Psychiatry 136:694-696.
13. Sohier, R. (1992). Feminism and nursing knowledge: The power of the weak. Nursing Outlook 40:62-66; 93.
14. Greenleaf, N. (1980). Sex-segregated occupations: Relevance for nursing. Advances in Nursing Science 2:23-29.
15. Levitin, T., Quinn, R., & Staines, G. (1975). Sex discrimination against the American working women. In: M. Mednick, S. Tangri, & L. Hoffman (Eds.), Women and Achievement. New York: Wiley and Sons. pp. 326-338.
16. Aiken, L., Blendon, R. & Rogers, D. (1981). The shortage of hospital nurses: A new perspective. American Journal of Nursing 81:1612-1618.

17. Brider, P. (1992). Salary gains slow as more RNs seek full-time benefits. American Journal of Nursing 92:34-40.
18. Edmunds, M. (1980). Non-clinical problems: Gender and the nurse practitioner role. Nurse Practitioner 5:42-43.
19. Schutzenhofer, K.K. (1988). The problem of professional autonomy in nursing. Health Care for Women International 9(2):93-106.
20. Mason, D.J., Backer, B.A. & Georges, A. (1991). Toward a feminist model for the empowerment of nurses. Image 23:72-77.

BIBLIOGRAPHY

Ashley, J.A. (1975). Nurses in American history: Nursing and early feminism. American Journal of Nursing 75:1465-1467.

Bullough, B. Barriers to the nurse practitioner movement: Problems of women in a women's field. Nursing Digest 6:49-54.

Bullough, B. & Bullough, V. (1978). Sex discrimination in health care. Nursing Outlook 23:40-45.

Clemons, B. (1971). Women's liberation and nursing. Historic interplay. AORN Journal 13:71-78.

Connors, D. (1980). Sickness unto death. Medicine as mythic, necrophilic and iatrogenic. Advances in Nursing Science 2:39-51.

Elliott, E.A. (1990). The discourse of nursing: A case of silencing. Nursing Health Care 11:539-543.

Felton, G. (1978). On women, networks, patronage and sponsorship. Image 10:58-59.

Ferguson, K.E. (1984). The Feminist Case Against Bureaucracy. Philadelphia: Temple University Press.

Heide, W.S. (1985). Feminism for the Health of It. Buffalo, NY: Margaretdaughters.

Heide, W.S. (1973). Nursing and women's liberation: A parallel. American Journal of Nursing 73:824-827.

Helgesen, S. (1992). Feminism and nursing. Revolution 2:50-57; 135.

Lovell, M. (1981). Silent but perfect "partners": Medicine's use and abuse of women. Advances in Nursing Science 3:25-40.

Muff, J. (Ed.) (1982). Socialization, Sexism, and Stereotyping: Women's Issues in Nursing. St. Louis, MO: C.V. Mosby.

Roland, C. (1977). The insidious bias of medical language. Nursing Digest 5:51-55.

Vance, C. (1979). Women leaders. Modern day heroines or societal deviants. Image 11:37-41.

Wheeler, C.E. & Chinn, P.L. (1984). Peace and Power: A Handbook of Feminist Process. 2nd ed. New York: National League for Nursing.

4

Power and Nursing: Need for a Paradigm of Empowerment*

Introduction

The word "power" has many connotations. It commonly implies an ability to control others by virtue of one's authority or to sway or influence others towards one's own viewpoint. Nurses are the only authorities who can speak for the profession of nursing when issues of role delineation, nursing actions, or nursing outcomes are in question.

Power can also be viewed as a capability for action as in the ability to perform or produce. The advanced practitioner gains access to this type of power through education and experience and through identifying resources which can be mobilized and brought to bear upon a particular situation to affect a desired outcome (1).

The latent power inherent in the professional nursing role should be capitalized upon in order to help shape the future directions of the health system and nursing's role in it. The advanced practitioner must learn to identify aspects of personal and professional power and to use this power to her/his advantage and in collaborating with nursing peers

---
*With Pauline F. Hebert, Ph.D.

within the profession to further the public and political image of nursing as an autonomous entity.

The Roots of Powerlessness

The roots of powerlessness in the profession today can be partially traced to nurses' socialization in traditional female roles and the profession's relations with physicians and hospital administrators. Before professional autonomy can be achieved, nurses need to understand nursing's historical ties to the system that has held them powerless (2).

Nursing education had its genesis in hospitals under the dominion of physicians. Fry maintains that, as a result, the nurse became fused to the hospital and physician in a dependency state (2). The fact that hospitals and physicians *needed* nurses and were dependent upon them to function was rarely overtly acknowledged by nurses and certainly was never capitalized on by them to develop a position of equality or interdependency with the medical profession.

Florence Nightingale attributed *all* successful recoveries to the ministrations of the "proper" nurses. When Nightingale arrived at Scutari in 1855, the death rate for sick and wounded soldiers averaged an alarming forty-two percent; under her management and the resultant sanitary improvements and nursing care, the death rate dropped to two percent in six months' time (3). In 1976, in Los Angeles and Bogota, Columbia, the death rate dropped eighteen percent in the former city and thirty-five percent in the latter city when physicians in both areas were on strike (4). From these statistical examples it would seem that Nightingale was more right than wrong as to who is dependent upon whom.

The slow erosion of nursing's power began in 1885 when Clara Weeks Shaw added qualifiers to nurses' independence. Shaw delineated the duties that nurses owed to physicians and stated that the recovery of the patient, in *some* instances, was more dependent on nursing than medical skill (5).

In the early nineteen hundreds, Bertha Harmer linked the entire profession of nursing to medicine rather than viewing nursing as a free-standing autonomous profession (6). As recently as the 1960s, some nursing leaders continued to espouse nursing's dependency.

Orlando conceptualized recipients of nursing care as being under medical care or supervision (7). In this instance, a nursing author explicitly stated that the client belonged to the physician. Is it any wonder then that medicine is viewed as possessing more power than nursing? Since the time of Florence Nightingale, a long history of subservience to and dependency on physicians can be documented, a history which must now, at last, be left behind in order to further nursing's efforts in meeting its goals. Ashley accurately pinpointed the difficulties when she made the observation that the powerlessness of the profession today resulted from the ways in which nurses used, misused, and abused their power (or failed to use it at all) as well as from the system in which nursing developed (8). Fry states that, as a profession, all nurses have to begin the process of divorcing themselves from those aspects of history which hold them back from independence and professional autonomy, thereby creating a proud legacy for the next generation of nurses (2).

Power as Influence

Within the profession of nursing there are many nurses who possess a great deal of latent power. Those in managerial positions, those who teach, and those who provide direct patient care are all in positions in which they can exert a great deal of power. Why then is this latent power not tapped? Why do most nurses feel powerless? Viewing power in action and analyzing aspects which influence one's ability to identify and use power can assist practitioners to mobilize their own strengths.

Since Florence Nightingale, few if any nurses have risen to a position of public power within society. This is not to imply that the nursing profession has not had its influential leaders nor that power has not been exerted on societies by nurses. Rather, efforts by nurses, when undertaken, have been exerted by collectives of individuals and not by loners. Nightingale, perhaps, stands alone, epitomizing the nurse leader waging a battle singlehandedly. Nightingale was responsible for significant organizational reforms within the army, the government, and the educational system. How many other nurses could boast of such broad and diverse achievements affecting complex organizations in society? "One of the world's most inspired and inspirational people, Florence Nightingale knew what she wanted to accomplish in her life and set out to do so, leaving a heritage rarely surpassed and seldom approximated in the history of women and of nations" (9).

One reason that nursing's power base has remained weak is that power tends to be associated with males and "men will go to extraordinary lengths to invent power structures...to deprive successful women of their autonomy" (10). Nursing's movement toward autonomy was thwarted when hospital administrators and physicians realized their dependence on nurses; this need was quickly expressed as a need to exert control over nurses (11). Florence Nightingale was astute enough to recognize the need men have to exert power over women and the threat that a competent woman presents to them. But she used this knowledge to her advantage.

Nightingale capitalized on other persons' influential ties, involving them in her causes and convincing them that her causes were to their benefit. Her reforms were carried out by men she personally inspired (9). Perhaps it is also significant that, at the time, England had a queen rather than a king, a queen who personally espoused some of Nightingale's reform measures. Power is influence and Nightingale developed the art of influence to perfection.

Power as Ability

Professional ability is dependent upon education and experience. The persistent fusion of many nurses to the hospital organization prevents many of them from seeing the need or value of advanced education. Many of these nurses are unwilling to augment their knowledge by a return to formal educational programs due to a sense of loyalty to the "parental" hospital system (2). Of even greater significance is the obvious lack of financial rewards once higher education credentials are attained. For men, education is usually directly correlated with income, social position, and occupational power. This is not necessarily so for females and, in particular, for nurses. McCarthy states that "...something is terribly wrong when experienced nurses, professionals who have worked full time for nearly twenty uninterrupted years on the staffs of hospitals and as university faculty members while putting themselves through graduate school are worth only forty cents an hour more than unlicensed graduates straight out of school.... In fact, in any other field, no one with those credentials would be working for an hourly wage'' (12). Because of this, many excellent nurses with advanced education have fled from hospital settings into other fields of endeavor such as academe, only to find inequities there also. In university settings, women on faculties, including those in schools of nursing, despite having in their possession all of the necessary academic credentials, are paid lower salaries for equivalent rank and/or responsibilities than males (13, 14).

Hospitals are the major focal point for professional nursing activities, employing sixty-six percent of all nurses in practice today (15). And, according to Lieb, ''...it is in such institutions [as hospitals] that domination by male authority is most obvious'' (11), a sentiment echoed by Muller and Cocotas (16).

Medical and hospital administration authorities have resisted and opposed baccalaureate nursing education since it was first proposed, for they understood how this would weaken their ability to maintain control of nurses (11). The lack of financial reimbursement for higher education credentials is only a manifestation of this resistance; the very fact that both groups continue to reap great financial profits while maintaining their secure power base at the expense of nurses should cause an American woman to feel some sense of outrage since it persists in a day touted as an age of equal opportunity.

Nightingale advocated ongoing education as a lifetime endeavor, stating that "no system can endure that does not march," and "...to stand still is to have gone back" (17).

"Nightingale was an accomplished linguist, informed in the arts, mathematics and statistics, well-read in philosophy and history, and perceptive about politics, economics and government. She exercised her eager and keen intelligence constantly as she furthered her inquiry into her own varied interests, which included religion, philosophy, land-use systems, liberty, freedom, social conditions and institutions" (9).

In the creation of Nightingale's school for nurses, she founded a one-year program which would prepare nurses for health maintenance, prevention of disease, detection of illness, and care of the sick (3). But even a Nightingale had episodes of intellectual darkness as when she simultaneously endorsed university education for women in general while she opposed the same educational preparation for nurses, perhaps because she failed to correlate her own superior accomplishments with her excellent educational preparation (9).

Power as Strength

Strength derives from a strong self-concept. A strong self-concept can be linked to a high level of motivation and success in one's career. Horner found that women demonstrate a need to avoid success and that, in particular, this avoidance behavior is aroused in women for whom success is a real possibility. The most competent women "when faced with a conflict between their feminine image and expressing their competencies or developing their abilities and interests, adjust their behaviors to their internalized sex-role stereotypes" (18). Sex-role stereotypes deliver messages which say that women have difficulty making decisions and are unable to act as leaders (19). Such messages affect women's self-concept, planting seeds of doubt about their ability to use their strength and power. Recent work by Veeder (21) refutes stereotypes of women as poor decision makers.

One of the better strategies for countering the effects of sex-role stereotyping is to identify one's personal skills and abilities as well as one's weaknesses and shortcomings. Knowing when one has the expertise to address a problem and identifying when external resources might be needed can facilitate success. Power can never be achieved without taking risks. It is of vital importance to analyze whether success or failure is most probable. Repeated failures influence one's self-concept, but a repertoire of repeated successes strengthens one's confidence in taking future risks.

Florence Nightingale demonstrated an ability to know when she needed to use external resources to implement her ideas and reforms.

Not only did she collaborate and consult with other influential persons to achieve her reforms, she also gathered statistics and facts to substantiate her opinions and recommendations. When she addressed an issue, she presented written material which was lucid and graphic so that her conclusions were unmistakable; she did not leave it to chance that her suggestions would be transmitted in printed official reports. Instead, she privately published these reports and disseminated them directly to the British people. She used the public press, sending letters to editors and publishing lively treatises on necessary reform (9). Florence Nightingale's self-concept, rooted in an accurate assessment of her own abilities and her educational background, was, without a doubt, intact and seldom threatened by public opinion, rumor or sex-role stereotyping.

External Resources

In order to obtain and utilize power, the nurse must gain access to a number of external resources to add to his or her own strengths. The creation of a new journal, *Revolution. The Journal of Nurse Empowerment,* in 1992 is a step in the right direction.

In 1971, a group of nursing leaders, calling themselves Nurses for Political Action, met to develop strategies for increasing nursing's sphere of influence. In 1973, this group became known as N-CAP (National Coalition for Action in Politics), becoming the political arm of the American Nurses Association. N-CAP and state political action committees have had an active role in influencing public policy. Notably, N-CAP has voiced opinions on the Equal Rights Amendment and national health insurance. Membership in a political action group is a way in which nurses can actively exert power and influence on our future health care delivery systems.

The National Organization of Women (NOW) has its own nursing chapter called Nurses Now. Membership in such an organization not only helps to expand the nurse's power base but also helps women to band together for mutual achievements that transcend subgroup interests. Nurses at the state and national level of NOW are working to influence legislators on bills relating to third party reimbursement and prescription writing privileges for nurses in expanded roles.

Political success, such as the override of the 1975 Presidential veto of the Nurse Training Act, is evidence of the power nursing is capable of wielding when members combine their efforts. Political education, awareness of issues, and group membership can all help bury the image of nurses as powerless. Empowerment enables nurses to participate in actions and decision-making within a context that supports an equitable distribution of power. "Empowerment requires a commitment to connection between self and others, enabling individuals or groups to recognize their own strengths, resources and abilities to make changes in their personal and public lives" (20). It is a process of confirming one's self and nursing.

Summary

A selective analysis on some aspects of power has been presented along with an historical perspective on power in action as it was demonstrated by that powerful nurse, Florence Nightingale. This nurse and leader was one of the few British individuals who emerged from England's disaster in the Crimean War with an enhanced reputation (9).

A knowledge of history can help nurses decide for themselves which strengths of the profession should be capitalized upon and which limitations should be discarded.

Nurse practitioners and clinical specialists represent a small minority within the profession. To remain isolated from the profession at large can only bring powerlessness. Power can be strengthened by unifying and consolidating nursing factions so that numbers can become important and meaningful in influencing the outcome of issues which impact upon the profession.

REFERENCES

1. Claus, K.E. & Bailey, J.T. (1977). Power and Influence in Health Care. St. Louis, MO: C.V. Mosby.

2. Fry, P.W. (1977). The need to differentiate. American Journal of Nursing 77:1452-1454.
3. Dolan, J. (1983). Nursing in Society. A Historical Perspective, 15th ed. Philadelphia: W.B. Saunders.
4. Wallace, I., Wallenchinsky, D. & Wallace, A. (1981). Doctors may be harmful. The Hartford Courant Parade Magazine, Oct. 4, p.23.
5. Shaw, C.S.W. (1885). A Textbook of Nursing. New York: D. Appleton and Company.
6. Harmer, B. (1922). Textbook of the Principles and Practice of Nursing. New York: The MacMillan Company.
7. Orlando, I.J. (1961). The Dynamic Nurse-Patient Relationship. New York: G.P. Putnam's Sons.
8. Ashley, J.A. (1973). About power in nursing. Nursing Outlook 21:637-641.
9. Palmer, I.S. (1977). Florence Nightingale: Reformer, reactionary, researcher. Nursing Research 26:84-89.
10. Korda, M. (1975). Power: How to Get It. How to Use It. New York: Ballentine Books. p. 255.
11. Lieb, R. (1978). Power, powerlessness and potential nurses' role within the health care delivery system. Image 10:75-82.
12. McCarthy, P.A. (1981). To halt the traffic in nurses. Nursing Outlook 29:509.
13. Astin, H. & Bayer, A. (1975). Sex discrimination in academe. In: M. Mednick, S. Tangri, & L. Hoffman (Eds.), Women and Achievement. New York: John Wiley & Sons. pp. 372-395.
14. Conway, M.E. (1978). The acquisition and use of power in academia: A dean's perspective. Nursing Administration Quarterly 2:83-90.
15. Aiken, L., Blendon, R.J. & Rogers, D. (1981). The shortage of hospital nurses: A new perspective. American Journal of Nursing 81:1612-1618.
16. Muller, H.J. & Cocotas, C. (1988). Women in power: New leadership in the health industry. Health Care for Women International 9(2):63-82.
17. Dolan, J. op.cit., p. 169.
18. Horner, M.S. (1975). Toward an understanding of achievement-reiated conflicts in women. In: M. Mednick, S. Tangri, & L. Hoffman (Eds.), Women and Achievement. New York: John Wiley & Sons. pp. 206-220.

19. Broverman, I., Vogel, S. Broverman, D., Charkan, F. & Rosenkrantz, F. (1975). In: M. Mednick, S. Tangri, & L. Hoffman (Eds.), Women and Achievement. New York: John Wiley & Sons. pp. 32-47.
20. Mason, D.J., Backer, B.A.. & Georges, A. (1991). Toward a feminist model for the political empowerment of nurses. Image 23:72-77.
21. Veeder, N.W. (1992). Women's Decision-Making. Common Themes... Irish Voices. Westport, CT: Praeger.

BIBLIOGRAPHY

Allen, D. (1987). Professionalism, gender segregation of labor and the control of nursing. Women and Politics 6(3):1-24.
Ashley, J.A. (1980). Power in structured misogyny. Implications for the politics of care. Advances in Nursing Science 2:3-22.
Beck, C.T. (1982). The conceptualization of power. Advances in Nursing Science 4(2):1-17.
Bookman, A. & Morgen, S. (Eds.) (1988). Women and the Politics of Empowerment. Philadelphia: Temple University Press.
Brooten, D.A. (1984). Managerial Leadership in Nursing. Philadelphia: Lippincott.
French, M. (1985). Beyond Power. New York: Ballentine.
Hennig, M. & Jordan, A. (1977). The Managerial Woman. New York: Pocket Books.
Lynaugh, J.E. & Fagin, C.M. (1988). Nursing comes of age. Image 20(4):184-189.
Melosh, B. (1986). The Physician's Hand. Philadelphia: Temple University Press.
Salancik, G.R., Pfeffen, J. (1983). Who gets power - and how they hold onto it: A strategic model of power. In: J. Hackman, E. Lawler & L. Porter (Eds.). Perspectives on Behavior in Organizations. New York: McGraw Hill. pp. 417-429.
Sohier, R. (1992). Feminism and nursing knowledge: The power of the weak. Nursing Outlook 40:62-66; 93.
Trahey, J. (1978). On Women and Power. New York: Avon Books.
Zerwekh, J.V. (1992). The practice of empowerment and coercion by expert public health nurses. Image 24:101-105.

5
The Concept of Change

Introduction

Nurse practitioners and clinical nurse specialists have been called the mavericks and risk-takers of the profession. Certainly, they are often in prime positions to implement changes in health care delivery. They can also help to define for the public what nurses can offer to their clients and help to effect a change in the stereotyping of nurses (1). They can be instrumental in redefining priorities for the health care system by shifting the focus from illness to wellness and from medical care to health care. They can influence health care policy. Finally, they can help to restructure the system of reimbursement for care so as to recognize the expertise of all members of the health care team.

In order to bring about change, however, it is important to understand various change strategies. Selection of the appropriate strategy can influence the outcome of the process and help to assure not only that change occurs, but also that it is lasting (if it is meant to be).

Initiating Change

Change comes about as the result of goal setting or identifying a problem (2). Some stimulus must be present for change to occur. Change may be planned or unplanned. Planned changes are designed to improve living, working, or recreational conditions in some way (3). In general, changes in health care delivery are aimed at improving the quality of care. Changes may also be directed at improving the satisfaction of those who give care or the setting in which care occurs. Thus, change may be directed at any one or all of three domains: structure, process, and outcome.

Unplanned change is change that is not desired by those in power. The results may, therefore, be unpredictable and unintended. It should be mentioned, however, that unplanned change is not always negative and, in fact, may have some important benefits for those whom it affects (4). The unforeseen resignation of the nurse administrator of an ambulatory service may result in the hiring of a new person with exciting and revolutionary ideas with regard to nurses' roles in ambulatory care. A change from young families to older adults in a neighborhood will profoundly affect the kinds of health care services that are required.

Initiation of planned change requires acknowledging 1) that there is a problem to which a solution may be found, and 2) that change is necessary. Those who would argue that nursing is a closed system which still clings to outmoded traditions and procedures should recall how Florence Nightingale used her gift of leadership to fight the existing health care system and used all the political power she could muster to bring about change (5).

At the same time that we have been digging in our heels and resisting change in nursing, we have also been part of the dramatic changes within our profession over the past one hundred plus years. Nursing has witnessed profound changes in its structure, educational objectives, and practice since Nightingale initiated the transition to professional status. We have moved to learning-based education, the development of graduate programs, research, theory bases for practice, and new roles and specialties. It is evident that nurses have been involved in change across the decades. Nonetheless, resistance to change still occurs (6). It is incumbent upon the nurse who becomes a change agent to make a case for change and convince his or her peers that change will, in the long run, benefit both the client and the profession.

Because health care agencies and institutions are often very complex, an organizational analysis can be useful prior to initiating change (7). Such an analysis not only helps to clarify needed changes, but also helps to identify key players, driving and restraining forces, and the change strategies that might be most effective.

Nurses in Advanced Practice as Change Agents

Mauksch and Miller have identified three characteristics of change agents (8). The first of these is being a risk-taker. The very nature of the advanced practitioner's role implies that these nurses are willing to try new identities and take on new aspects of their practice and increased accountability.

Changes in identity and function occur when a nurse acquires the knowledge and skills to practice the new role of nurse practitioner or clinical specialist. Assuming the role requires a commitment to practice that a basic program has usually not prepared one for. It may mean giving up stereotypic images of what a nurse is, does, and should be. Participating as a colleague on the health care delivery team may be a new experience. Every change agent must possess competence as a practitioner, skills in interpersonal relations, and a knowledge of nursing based on research findings and basic scientific information (8). As an organizational development consultant, a clinical nurse specialist or nurse practitioner may be in a prime position to help initiate change (9).

Theories of Change and Change Strategies

Kurt Lewin, the source of classical change theory, viewed change as occurring in three steps: unfreezing, moving, and refreezing. He also emphasized the need to identify those forces that support change

The Concept of Change

(driving forces) and those that mediate against it (restraining forces) (10). A number of other theorists who modified Lewin's theories are discussed in Welch's article on change (11).

Chin and Benne in their classic volume on change describe three types of basic strategies: empirical-rational, normative-re-educative, and power-coercive (12). The rest of this chapter will examine these three categories for their application to the change process in nursing.

Empirical-Rational Strategies

Empirical-rational strategies are based on the assumption that people are rational beings. The development of basic research in nursing and the dissemination of its results through education and the literature is one example of this kind of strategy. Nurses in programs preparing them for advanced practice roles may thus be educated to practice in a particular model and incorporate the values of their preceptors.

Those selected for key positions in organizations affect the way nursing is practiced. A nursing director of a student health service who is strongly committed to implementing the role of nurse practitioner in primary care delivery can effect change in the way nurses are utilized. An elite corps of nurse practitioners may be utilized to demonstrate the role.

Using those who are experts in implementing a nursing model for practice as consultants or staff can be one strategy to effect change from a disease-oriented medical approach to a health-oriented nursing model. Another strategy is to use experts in communication and semantics to assure that people in the organization communicate more effectively. Human relations training techniques can be used to improve both intra- and interdisciplinary staff communications.

Normative-Re-educative Strategies

These strategies are premised on the belief that humans are active beings and as such will seek to satisfy their needs and impulses (13). Humans are also social beings affected by the norms of their culture as well as by internalized beliefs and values. To occur, then, change must involve the

habits and values of the individuals and norms of the society (13).
Some of the strategies under this category involve use of change agents to involve the client or system in working out changes. The change agent must be a consultant, researcher, friend, or therapist to the client. In nursing, curriculum consultants may be utilized to effect change in an educational system. A clinical nurse specialist can be hired to demonstrate health care delivery for clients and providers. This person's success will be based partly on an ability to collaborate with clients and others in delivering care. For change to last, beliefs about advanced practitioners must be explored and value conflicts must be worked through.

Psychotherapy is another example of a normative-re-educative strategy. Nurses are primary therapists for clients. There is also a movement toward more nurse involvement in primary care in mental health settings. One of the objectives of therapy can be to help clients or families develop better problem-solving and coping capabilities.

Nurses in primary care often use strategies to help individuals, families, or groups achieve growth and maximize the biophysical and psychosocial aspects of development. Strategies may be utilized to effect behavior modification, to achieve developmental tasks, and to reach or maintain a higher level of health.

Staff development programs can be used to effect change in a system. Introducing and adopting problem-oriented records will involve normative-re-educative processes if the nurses have been educated to use more traditional methods of recording.

Power-Coercive Strategies

The use of power and coercion to bring about change is familiar to all of us. Nurses work in a system in which physicians have been treated as gatekeepers for that system. Traditional nurses' training stressed obedience, submission, and adherence to physicians' orders (14). Nurses have been the victims of power abuse rather than the users of power.

Using confrontation as one coercive strategy can be advantageous to nurses as a precursor to change (14). In some settings they may be grappling with role issues in relation to physicians. They may see themselves being used more as handmaidens than as colleagues in what is supposed to be a collaborative process of health care delivery. Planning is important if the strategy of confrontation is to be used positively. After using confrontation as a strategy to discuss issues, the outcomes should be evaluated (14).

Confrontation can be useful in effecting change when an advanced practice role is introduced. Nurses will have to use their expert power to implement the role; they may need to be confrontive in refusing to respond to physicians' expectations of subservience, such as demands to change the examining table paper, call in clients, or assist with procedures—unless these courtesies are mutual. For instance, one nurse manager used her coercive powers as a member of an executive committee responsible for an ambulatory clinic to enforce how her advanced practitioners were and were not to be utilized.

In order to effect change, coercion is sometimes necessary. In implementing a client education program, for example, it was necessary for one nurse manager to require all her advanced practitioners to participate. Left to volunteers, the program would have failed, as the same few individuals would have burned out quickly.

Political activism through lobbying at local, state, and national levels is another example of the use of coercive strategies. The power of our vote will influence the actions of those who represent us. Nurses also hold political offices and serve in high offices in the National Institutes of Health, the Health Resources and Services Administration, and other departments of the federal government. There they can use the influence of their positions to chart the course of health care policy making.

A power elite can be created in nursing as in other professions to affect the course of nursing practice and to effect change. The officers of the National League for Nursing and the American Nurses Association might be viewed by some as a power elite, as might the Council of Nurses in Advanced Practice of the American Nurses Association. Networking can be one way of connecting with the power elite of the profession (15).

Implementing Change

Goal/Problem Identification

The first step in implementing change is to delineate a goal clearly or identify the problem which has precipitated a need for change (16). Do we desire to bring about a change in attitudes? An alteration in physicians' perceptions of the role of the advanced practitioner is one example of an attitudinal change we might want to achieve. The change may be technical; for example, the use of fetal monitors on all clients in active labor. Teaching clients self-examination of the breast is an informational change and, hopefully, a behavioral one as well. Adoption of the use of a problem-oriented system of record keeping necessitates a procedural change. Reorganization of the physical layout of a clinical unit would constitute a structural or environmental change. Implementing care in a unit with labor, delivery, recovery, and postpartum rooms (LDRP) might be a role for a perinatal clinical nurse specialist and involve structural and procedural changes, and perhaps attitudinal and behavioral changes for staff members.

Recipients of Change

The recipients of change must be identified. Will the change affect staff, clients, the environment, the system as a whole, a subsystem, or some or all of these? How is the change to be introduced to those whom it will affect?

Sources of Resistance

Identifying possible sources of resistance is helpful in selecting change strategies as well as in anticipating how the process will progress. Is the climate conducive to change? (17) Will the change pose a real threat to anyone's job? Will the choice of change agent generate resistance? How best can the change be implemented so as to preserve the integrity of the system as a whole as well as the self-esteem, competence, and autonomy of those affected by the change? Where does the real power lie in the agency? How can the cooperation of this person or these persons be engaged?

Strategies

Strategies to be used to implement the change must be appropriate not only for the type of change to be accomplished but also for the system. For example, coercive strategies may be acceptable when it has been decided to substitute one type of examination gloves for another; in this case, a simple memo to all those affected would suffice. When choosing a new nurse manager, however, similar tactics will probably elicit a strong response, and careful planning is necessary in selecting and planning the strategies to be used since the change is likely to affect others significantly. Those who will be affected by a significant change need to be informed about the process and the goals(s) and educated for any new processes, procedures, or technology. Plans need to be made for any administrative adjustments that will occur as a result of the change or in order to support the project.

If possible, the change should be tested on a small scale before instituting it agency-wide. Introducing an advanced practice nurse into the pediatrics clinic may be followed by hiring advanced practitioners for geriatric and young adult services if the evaluations are positive. A new type of examination glove can be tried in one clinic before they are purchased for the entire outpatient service. Evaluating the pilot project will help to iron out any kinks before the change is adopted agency-wide (2). A psychiatric liaison nurse might begin work with a surgical unit and then, based on feedback, offer her/his services to medical, obstetrical, and other units.

Evaluating Change

Once a change has been effected, evaluation of the change and its effectiveness should occur. Beginning with a goal or objectives gives one criteria by which to evaluate the change. Has it accomplished the goal? If not, why? Are the means appropriate to the end? How have those affected responded to the change? (2). If advanced practitioners are hired for ambulatory service and, as a result, other staff resign, is the end worth the means?

Change should be assessed as to its effectiveness, efficiency, and satisfaction for all those involved. Longevity is an index of the effectiveness of change. Efficiency can be measured in time, energy, and dollars. Change is effective if it proves to be more acceptable, pleasing, and comfortable than the original structure, process, or outcome to all those whom it affects (2).

Last, it is important to report the change. Disseminating information about the change and evaluating the process and outcome can be helpful not only to those directly affected by the change but also to sponsors of the change (government, private foundation, agency administration), researchers and students, change agents in other settings, and colleagues in the profession (18). Internal and external communication about the change can be appropriate. Publication should be considered (18). One might say that until communication about a change has occurred, the process is not complete.

Summary

The nurse practitioner and the clinical nurse specialist roles underline the potential for a strong contribution to and strong leadership for new models for delivering health care.

Change is inevitable as the present system is assaulted by technological advances, consumer demands for accountability and cost effectiveness, cost escalation, the women's movement, and changes within the profession affecting the images and roles of nurses. We have the power to be change agents, to affect the delivery of health care in our practices and to effect change for the system as a whole. "Planned change is part of today's nurses' leadership roles" (11). It is, therefore, an integral part of the roles of the nurse practitioner and clinical nurse specialist.

REFERENCES

1. Carr, E.M. (1982) Networking: A resource for change. The Nurse Practitioner 7:32-34.
2. Stevens, B.J. (1977) Management of continuity and change in nursing. Journal of Nursing Administration 7:26-31.
3. Mauksch, I.G. & Miller, M.H. (1981) Implementing Change in Nursing. St. Louis: C.V. Mosby. p. 20.

4. Ibid., p. 22.
5. Garant, C.A. (1978) The process of effecting change in nursing. Nursing Forum 17:152-167.
6. Mauksch, I.G. & Miller, M.H., op cit., p. 32.
7. Reddecliff, M., Smith, E.L. & Ryan-Merritt, M. (1989). Organizational analysis: Tool for the clinical nurse specialist. Clinical Nurse Specialist 3(3):133-136.
8. Mauksch, I.G. & Miller, M.H., op. cit., pp. 33-34.
9. McDougall, G.J. (1987). The role of the clinical nurse specialist consultant in organizational development. Clinical Nurse Specialist 1(3):133-139.
10. Lewin, K. (1958) Group decision and social change. In: E. Maccoby (Ed.) Readings in Social Psychology (3rd ed.). New York: Holt, Rinehart and Winston.
11. Welch, L.B. (1979) Planned change in nursing: The theory. Nursing Clinics of North America 14:306-321.
12. Chin, R. & Benne, K.D. (1984) General strategies for effecting changes in human systems. In: W.G. Bennis, K.D. Benne & R. Chin (Eds.) The Planning of Change (4th ed.). Chicago: Holt, Rinehart and Winston.
13. Ibid., p. 31.
14. Smoyak, S.A. (1974) The confrontation process. American Journal of Nursing 74:1632-1635.
15. Fain, J.A. & Viau, P. (1989). Networking: A strategy for strengthening the role of the clinical nurse specialist. Clinical Nurse Specialist 3(1), 29-31.
16. Bailey, J.T. & Claus, K.E. (1975) Decision Making in Nursing Tools for Change. St. Louis: C.V. Mosby, p. 20.
17. Hofing, A.L., McGugin, M.B. & Merkel, S.I. (1979) The importance of maintenance in implementing change: An experience with problem-oriented recording. Journal of Nursing Administration 9:43-48.
18. Mauksch, I.G. & Miller, M.H., op. cit., pp. 158-159.

BIBLIOGRAPHY
Brooten, D.A. (1984). Managerial Leadership in Nursing. Philadelphia: J.B. Lippincott.
Jernigan, D.K. (1988). Human Resource Management in Nursing. Norwalk, CT: Appleton & Lange.
Roberts, L.R. (1987). Clinical nurse specialist: Line or staff using Lewin's field theory to resolve the issue. Clinical Nurse Specialist 1(1):39-44.

6

Legal Aspects of Advanced Practice

Introduction

The first nurse registration statutes were passed in 1903 in New York, North Carolina, New Jersey, and Virginia. By 1923, all states had nurse registration acts on their books. In 1938, the second phase of such legislation began with New York's mandatory practice act to define two levels of nurses: registered and practical (1).

Today, all state statutes relating to nursing contain a definition of nursing, requirements for licensure and for endorsing those licensed in other states, and rules and regulations governing the licensure processes and the board of examiners. The key to practice is the definition of nursing. This is especially important for nurses whose practice encroaches on what has traditionally been hallowed medical turf. In this chapter, we will examine some legal aspects of the roles, including practice acts, credentialing, and malpractice issues.

Nurse Practice Acts

In 1955, the American Nurses Association proposed a model definition of nursing for state nurse practice acts. In part, this definition reads: "The practice of professional nursing means the performance for compensation of any act in the observation, care, and counsel of the ill, injured, or infirm, or in the maintenance of health or prevention of illness of others...the foregoing shall not be deemed to include acts of diagnosis or prescription of therapeutic or corrective measures" (2).

Many states utilized this definition in their acts. In 1970, acknowledging advanced practice roles, the American Nurses' Association suggested that states might wish to consider modifying their definitions if they appeared too restrictive. To that end, the following definition was proposed: "A professional nurse may also perform such additional acts, under emergency or other special conditions, which may include special training, as are recognized by the medical and nursing professions as proper to be performed by a professional nurse under such conditions, even though such acts might otherwise be considered diagnosis and prescription" (2). Clearly, this definition spells out the need for special preparation while at the same time recognizing the overlap with medicine that delivery of care by advanced practitioners may require. In 1971 Idaho became the first state to incorporate advanced practice into its definition of nursing (3).

The 1971 report to the Secretary of Health, Education, and Welfare indicated that state licensure laws were not perceived as obstacles to extending roles for nurses as those roles were conceived by the authors of the report. The recommendation was made to consider licensure and certification and develop a model law which might be applicable nationwide (4).

A survey of state boards of nursing in 1980 revealed that fifteen states have retained a traditional definition of nursing similar or identical to the one proposed as a model in 1955 by ANA.

In 1982, a new Nurse Practice Act was signed into law in Rhode Island. In part, this law states that "The assessment of an individual's health status, identification of health care needs, determination of health care goals . . . and the development of a plan of nursing care to

achieve these goals" are part of the role of the professional nurse (5).
The National Council of State Boards of Nursing published a new model nursing practice act in 1982. The model definition of practice is: "The 'practice of nursing' means assisting individuals or groups to maintain or attain optimal health throughout the life process by assessing their health status, establishing a diagnosis, planning and implementing a strategy of care to accomplish defined goals, and evaluating responses to care and treatment" (6).

Following these examples, nurses in other states have examined their nurse practice acts, as well as who holds regulatory control over advanced nursing practice. Alaskan nurses have been successful in updating their nurse practice act to include a definition of an advanced nurse practitioner, as well as regaining control over all levels of nursing (7). In Ohio, a new nursing practice act has been passed; included in the definition of professional nursing is recognition of an advanced nursing practice title (8). In 37 states, advanced practice as a nurse practitioner and/or clinical nurse specialist is covered under specific regulations in the nurse practice act to define advanced practice under their state boards of nursing. In 8 states, advanced practitioners practice under a broad nurse practice act, and in 6 states, nurse practitioners are regulated by the state boards of nursing and medicine — in Pearson's words, "an outrageous barrier to practice!" (9). Some states are struggling with updated definitions of nursing practice that will be included in their nurse practice acts as they are revised, and some states have very restrictive practice acts for advanced practitioners (10).

Special Legislation for Expanded Nursing Practice

A number of states are considering or have passed legislation on prescription writing for nurse practitioners. By the end of 1980, thirteen states had experimental or functional regulations whereby nurses can write prescriptions (11). Mechanisms include requirements for continuing education, limitations on the types of prescriptions, special courses and examinations, and notification of medical and nursing boards as to practice sites (12).

A study of the prescription writing practices of nurse practitioners in Michigan revealed that they make effective and appropriate use of such privileges. The study supports the continuation of such practices (13). Other analyses of nurses' prescription writing activities support the safety of their practices (14, 15).

By 1993, 43 states (including the District of Columbia) had granted prescription writing privileges to advanced practitioners. In some of these states, the law specifies nurse practitioners; in others, it specifies nurses in advanced practice roles, including clinical nurse specialists. The enabling legislation also frequently spells out additional preparation and/or the use of protocols, and/or an official formulary. In 21 of these states, dependent statutory regulations exist, and in 22, independent prescribing authorities (16). Some states limit nurses' prescriptive authority under one or more areas: category of clients served by advanced practice nurses, and drug schedules and classifications needed in the nursing specialty practice (17).

In the few states where a prescribing law does not yet exist, many nurses in advanced practice are writing prescriptions on presigned pads, writing prescriptions and then having the physician sign them, distributing stock medications, calling in prescriptions to pharmacies, and/or writing a prescription and signing the nurse practitioner or clinical nurse specialist or nurse midwife's and physician's name (18).

Trends identified in state nurse practice acts include increasing physician involvement through rule setting by joint boards, mandatory use of protocols, policies, procedures, and standardized rules prepared by employing agencies or physicians, and requiring a written agreement between nurse and physician. It is also evident that more states are mandating education and/or practice requirements for expanded roles and certification by a national certification board or by the state itself (16).

Authorization for advanced practice varies among the states. In 37 states nurse practitioners, certified nurse midwives, nurse anesthetists, and/or clinical nurse specialists are regulated by the Board of Nursing and specific regulations exist. Eight states have a broad nurse practice act under which advanced practice is regulated, and in six others advanced practice is regulated by both the Board of Nursing and the Board of Medicine. Some of the 37 nurse practice acts with specific advanced practice regulations name advanced practitioners by title; others use the title "advanced practitioner of nursing (APN)." Trends on a national level include moves by states to tighten licensing laws, increase professional accountability, require a master's degree for advanced practice roles, set national practice standards, use national certification as a credentialing mechanism, have stronger licensure laws and boards, put consumers on boards, develop equivalency examinations for educational programs and occupations, and put in place mechanisms to insure provider mobility as well as increased accountability (19). Even through these trends were identified 26 years ago, they continue to this day!

Federal law affects many aspects of advanced practice. Economic aspects are discussed in Chapter Ten. A national health insurance plan would dramatically change delivery of health care and the roles of nurses in advanced practice. The Nursing Home Reform Law of 1987 expanded the authority of nurse practitioners and clinical nurse specialists in the care of nursing home residents, including prescription authority (20). In late 1992, the American Nurses Association announced success in lobbying the Drug Enforcement Administration to reconsider regulations limiting nurses' prescribing of controlled substances (21). These are but two examples of federal legislation affecting practice. Specialty organizations and state nurses associations keep members apprised of legislation on the state and federal levels and lobby on behalf of nurses.

It is clear that the creation of advanced practice roles for nurses has had an impact on how we choose, in a legal sense, to define nursing practice. It is equally clear that the roles have incited dissension about the scope of practice, not only within the profession but with other health care providers, most notably physicians. If we are to retain control of our practice and how it is to be defined, we will have to become more active politically.

Certification and Credentialing

National Certification

In 1973, the American Nurses' Association announced its intention to initiate a pilot program for national certification to recognize excellence in nursing practice. The first 191 nurses were certified in 1974 and honored in a formal ceremony in January, 1975 (22).

In the ANA bylaws adopted at the 1976 convention, each practice division is charged with providing "recognition of professional achievement and excellence in its area of concern" (23). The original intention, which was to recognize excellence, yielded to pressures by consumers, third party payers, and others, so that by 1978, the year in which ANA voted to fund the certification process for two years, the purposes had expanded. Dr. Mauksch, chairperson of the Interdivisional Council on Certification, identified these purposes as: assurance of quality beyond basic licensure; identification of nurses who may be directly reimbursable for services; and recognizing achievement and quality of practice (17).

Certification in 1978 included the following specialties: maternal-gynecological nursing; psychiatric/mental health nursing; clinical specialist in psychiatric and mental health nursing; adult and family nurse practitioners; community health nursing; gerontological nursing; pediatric nurse practitioner (ambulatory); clinical specialist in medical-surgical nursing; and medical-surgical nurse. By that same year, 1,350 nurses had been certified. In 1979, school nurse-practitioner, nursing of acute and chronically ill children, and high-risk perinatal nursing were added (23).

As of 1992, ANA listed more than 84,000 nurses who had achieved ANA certification in 22 categories. Examinations are now available for 20 clinical and two administrative areas (24).

In 1980, by mutual consent with ANA, the Nurses' Association of the American College of Obstetricians and Gynecologists took over the credentialing of obstetric/gynecologic nurse practitioners, inpatient obstetric nurses, and neonatal intensive care nurses. By 1993, this group changed its name to the National Certification Corporation for the Obstetric, Gynecologic, and Neonatal Nursing Specialties, and had added neonatal nurse practitioner, low risk neonatal nurse, high risk obstetric nurse, ambulatory women's health care nurse, and reproductive endocrinology/infertility nurse (25). The American Nurses Association through the American Nurses Credentialing Center continues to certify those groups listed for 1978 and 1979 with the exception of maternal/newborn nurses, and now requires a master's degree for its five nurse practitioner and five clinical specialist certification programs. (24). Occupational health is a new component of community health. The American Board for Occupational Health Nurses certifies nurses for this area of practice. The American College of Nurse Midwives continues to certify nurse midwives who are graduates of the programs which it accredits. The American Association of Nurse Anesthetists certifies nurse anesthetists in a manner similar to that of the ACNM. The National Association of Pediatric Nurse Associates and Practitioners (NAPNAP) sponsors, together with the American Academy of Pediatrics, the National Qualifying Examinations for Pediatric Nurse Practitioners/Associates.

According to 1988 figures, there were 16,931 nurse anesthesists in active practice (26). In 1990, there were 4,200 nurse midwives. In addition, by 1991, the American Nurses Association listed 28,412 currently certified nurse practitioners and clinical nurse specialists (24), and the National Certification Corporation had 31,241 nurses listed, 15% or more of whom are ob/gyn or neonatal nurse practitioners (27). Additionally, NAPNAP had several thousand certified pediatric nurse practitioners and there are additional certifying organizations. However, nurses do hold certification in more than one area. Furthermore, almost two dozen nursing organizations and several interdisciplinary associations are now involved in credentialing nurses. Questions remain in spite of the deluge of certification possibilities. One article raised the important query: "Is it a passing fad or a lasting trend?" (28).

Several important and troubling questions are raised by the plethora of credentialing bodies and examinations. Credentialing does not have a uniform meaning, and the criteria for certification and recertification vary (29). Educational requirements to sit for a certification examination range from holding a license to practice as an RN to a minimum of a master's degree for some advanced practice certification (30). The cost of certification to the candidate is considerable, and achievement of certification sometimes goes unrecognized by the employer. In Beecroft and Papenhausen's words, "... the recognition of advanced specialty practice through certification is an issue that has been debated without resolution" (31). These authors go on to raise important questions: what is the purpose, who should be certified, who should benefit, who should control professional practice, who should set standards of care and what qualifications must such an individual have, what is the place of graduate education for certification, and should certification be voluntary or mandatory? At this writing, two organizations of specialty groups in nursing are struggling with these issues: the National Federation of Specialty Nursing Organizations (NFSNO) and the National Organization Liaison Forum (NOLF) (31).

Another question raised by issues of certification and the broader topic of credentialing is what nurses are to be called who are credentialed beyond their basic nursing preparation that allowed them to sit for licensure and use the initials RN. Titling is a troublesome issue, as it involves not only professional but also public recognition of who nurses are and what differentiates who we are and how we practice; that is, what we are allowed to do under nurse practice acts and what the public has a right to expect from us. In her landmark work on specialization in nursing, Styles (32) urged us as a profession to empower ourselves through self-regulation. The 1990s promise to urge us forward as the nation considers reform of health care and the place of advanced practice in that reform.

State Certification

In recent times, some states have elected to institute their own methods for certifying nurses for advanced practice and state this in their statutes. Others recognize national certification as part of the process of obtaining an advanced practice license as a nurse practitioner and/or clinical nurse specialist. Two states require a master's for certain advanced practitioners. Seventeen states have chosen to recognize certification by a national certifying body and state this in their statutes. Thirteen states have adopted a different format requiring state certification. This means that one must provide documentation of educational preparation for advanced practice and meet other statutory requirements such as a written agreement with a physician, standing orders and protocols [in some states evaluated by the licensing board(s)], and so on.

As of 1988, most states plus the District of Columbia and the Virgin Islands had basic laws mentioning the practice of nurse-midwives. Of these, several grant a state certificate (33). Additionally, several states certify nurse anesthetists.

National Credentialing

In 1976, ANA launched a study on credentialing. Numerous nursing organizations, the state boards, and the USPHS's Division of Nursing were represented in developing the proposal for the study (34). The study was reported out of committee in January 1979. In an extensive report, the committee delineated its fourteen principles of credentialing and set forth position statements on definitions of nursing, entry into practice, educational mobility, control and cost of credentialing, accountability, and competence. The committee then went on to recommend a model for credentialing in nursing in the form of a national credentialing center (25). A plan for follow-up of the study was handed over to ANA and the many cooperating groups (36). The response of the National League for Nursing to the credentialing study was to take no formal position for or against the recommendations and to note that many questions remain unanswered (27). ANA's Commission on Organizational Assessment and Renewal (COAR) studied a variety of models for ANA and other specialty nursing organizations. A most important part of this work was consideration of the relationship between ANA's certification programs and those of other nurse certifying bodies. In the final report, creating a separate credentialing center for nursing was recommended, following external standards for credentialing agencies. ANA has established a separate center, but it is one of many credentialing and certifying groups for nursing (38).

The credentialing report from Health, Education, and Welfare issued in 1977 suggests further investigation of the concept of certification of health professionals at the national level (39). As of 1993, no plan has been developed or implemented, although it would be consistent with the federal trends discussed earlier in the chapter. Whether the Public Health Service will be content with actions on the part of professional organizations such as ANA in the credentialing area or choose to enact federal mandates remains to be seen.

In 1982, a meeting was held of the National Specialty Nursing Certifying Organizations. The agenda focused on the meaning of certification and suggestions for the future of certification programs. Those attending included ANA, NAACOG Certification Corporation, American Board of Occupational Health Nurses, American College of Nurse Midwives, Division of Examiners, and NAPNAP (40). By 1987, two national nursing organizations had been formed: the National Federation of Specialty Nursing Organizations (NFSNO) and the Nursing Organization Liaison Forum (NOLF). Both have among their concerns certification (41). These groups continue to struggle with issues of credentialing and certification, having received support through Macy Foundation funding.

Issues of Malpractice for Nurses in Advanced Practice

In this age of litigation, it is not surprising that nurses are concerned about their legal status and vulnerability. Nurses can be and are being sued. However, after 18 months of data collection by the National Practitioner Data Bank (September 1990—February 1992), there is encouraging news. The rate of malpractice payments for nurses in advanced practice (per 1,000 practitioners) nurse anesthetists was 6.7: for nurse midwives it was 5.5, and for nurse practitioners it was 1.0 and 0.2 for registered nurses. (42). These figures compared with a rate of 32.2 for allopathic physicians.

Issues for malpractice suits usually rest on what is "reasonably prudent" for a practitioner to do whose background is similar to that of the individual being sued. Some specific questions are raised in the case of nurses in advanced practice. Who will the "expert" witness be — a nurse or a physician? By whom are policies and practices written? Does the literature reflect well-researched practice? Are the professional standards for practice (ANA and others) unrealistic ideals or are they attainable? What will be the standard of care for advanced practice? Some important questions have been raised about legal dangers of written protocols and standards. If the standards are unreasonable, they may make the practitioner vulnerable (43). Patients' rights and informed consent are also critical issues (44, 45).

As nurses become more vulnerable to suits, protection is important. Nurses choosing to protect their practices with malpractice insurance need to familiarize themselves with the risks covered in the policy, the amount of coverage provided, and the conditions spelled out (46, 47).

It is important to understand the difference between an occurrence-based professional liability insurance policy and a claims-made policy. An occurrence-based policy provides coverage for any incident which *occurred* during the time the policy was in effect. A claims-made policy covers the nurse for any suit *filed* while the policy is in effect (48).

Nurses should consider individual policies even if they are covered by blanket institutional policies. It is important to explore all sources of policies. Group policies available through professional organizations may be cheaper, but it is important to scrutinize the coverage and compare carefully. State insurance laws will guide you as to who is issuing professional liability policies.

Be sure to check whether a policy will cover your practice as a nurse practitioner or clinical nurse specialist whatever your setting and mode of practice. Does the policy cover all your professional activities? Does it duplicate other insurance you may have? What are the exclusions? Are they important to your practice? What are the premiums? Remember, these are tax deductible as a professional expense. Will the policy pay a reasonable amount? Is there a limit on the amount per incident or on total coverage? If so, is it adequate? How is payment made for a claim? Does it cover legal fees? Can claims be settled without your consent? Must the claim be determined to be valid before a legal defense can begin? What are your responsibilities as the insured party? (49). Given the malpractice insurance crisis for advanced practice of the 1980s, nurses must be well informed and should participate in legislative activity regarding malpractice insurance (50). Furthermore, they must assist in providing accurate data concerning liability claims (51, 52).

In 1978, Senator Daniel K. Inouye of Hawaii introduced a bill to establish a no-fault federal malpractice compensation system. Health care professionals could subscribe. The intent was to curb the destructive forces present in the suit-conscious private enterprise system that pit providers and consumers against each other in the legal arena (53). To date, no such bill has been passed. This attempt, however, represents an important effort to call off the accelerating legal cold war between health care professionals and the clients they serve. Perhaps such a plan will be part of health care reform in the 1990s.

It is obvious that, if present trends continue, more and more persons will choose professions with fewer legal risks, even though the monetary rewards may be less. The cost of malpractice insurance for some medical specialties already dissuades many. Where the spiraling of the legal costs of health care will take us is not clear. What is evident is that the present obsession with malpractice litigation encourages defensive practice on the part of the professions, increases costs for clients and/or third party reimbursement programs, and undermines the fundamental trust relationship inherent in the caring professions.

Summary

The nurse in advanced practice needs to know about the legal aspects of her or his role. This includes knowing the legal definitions for practice, including state nurse practice acts and state and federal legislation affecting practice, being aware of the standards and scope of practice as defined by professional organizations and what these mean from a legal perspective for advanced practice, and paying attention to documents such as the Code for Nurses and the Patient's Bill of Rights. The nurse who can speak with authority about the role and what responsibilities it encompasses is in an optimal position to define that role. If she or he is unable to be articulate about what constitutes the advanced practice role, others may dictate what that role is to be (54).

REFERENCES

1. Bullough, B. (1976). Influences on role expansion. American Journal of Nursing 76:1476-1481.
2. Kelly, L.Y. (l974). Nursing practice acts. American Journal of Nursing 74:1310-1319.
3. Bellocq, J.A. (1988). Part I: Florida's nurse practitioner act —

defining practice. Florida Nursing Review 2(3):3.
4. Secretary's Committee to Study Extended Roles for Nurses (1971). Extending the Scope of Nursing Practice. Washington, DC: U.S. Government Printing Office.
5. Carroby, J.J. (Nov. 15, 1982). Governor's letter to health care professionals. State of Rhode Island and Providence Plantations, Executive Chamber.
6. The Model Nursing Practice Act. (1982). Chicago: The National Council of State of State Broads of Nursing, Inc.
7. Bertholf, C.B. (1986). Alaska implements new prescription regulations for advanced NPs. The Nurse Practitioner 11(4):10, 15-16.
8. Stallmeyer, J. (1985). NPs score victory in Massachusetts. Ohio introduces new npa. The Nurse Practitioner 10(6):15, 32.
9. Pearson, L.J. (1993). 1992-93 update: How each state stands on legislative issues affecting advanced nursing practice. The Nurse Practitioner 18(1):25.
10. Ibid., pp. 25-26.
11. An update on prescription privileges for nurse practitioners. (1980). Newsletter of the Council of Primary Health Care Nurse Practitioners 3:5.
12. Council Update. Wellness: Focus for the 80s. (Nov. 14, 1980). Philadelphia: American Nurses' Association Annual Conference for the Council of Primary Health Care Nurse Practitioners.
13. Munroe, D., Pohl, J., Gardner, H.H. & Bell, R.E. (1982). Prescribing patterns of nurse practitioners. American Journal of Nursing 82:1538-1542.
14. Mahoney, D.F. (1992). Nurse practitioners as prescribers: Past research trends and future study needs. The Nurse Practitioner 17(1):44; 47-48; 50-51.
15. Harkless, G.E. (1989). Prescriptive authority: Debunking common assumptions. The Nurse Practitioner 14(8),57-58; 60-61.
16. Pearson, L.J. (1993) op cit., p. 24.
17. Gunn, I.P., Tobin, M.H., Rupp, R.M. & Blumenreich, G.A. (1990). Nurses and prescriptive authority. Specialty Nursing Forum 2(1):1; 3-6.

18. Pearson, L.J. (1993). op cit., p. 25.
19. Copp, L.A. & Kelly, L.S. (1977). Legal factors. In: Primary Care in a Pluralistic Society: Impediments to Health Care Delivery. Kansas City, MO: American Academy of Nursing. pp. 35-40.
20. Mittelstadt, P. (1991). New rules expand role of NPs, CNSs. The American Nurse 23(10):10.
21. Mercer, M. (1992). DEA reconsider regulation on prescriptive authority. The American Nurse 24(9):13.
22. National certification. An idea that's here for good. (1981). The American Nurse 13:11.
23. ANA funds certification program for two years. New areas added. (1978). American Journal of Nursing 78:534-541.
24. American Nurses Credentialing Center Certification Catalog. (1990). Washington, DC: American Nurses Credentialing Center.
25. NCC Catalog. (1993). Chicago: The National Certification Corporation.
26. National Sample Survey of Registered Nurses. (1988). Washington, DC: US Department of Health and Human Services.
27. NCC News, August 1992, p. 2.
28. del Bueno, D. (1988). The promise and reality of certification. Image 20:208-211.
29. Knapp, J.E. (1990). Continuing competency: A search for clarification. Specialty Nursing Forum 3(2):1; 6-7.
30. Napier, A.H. (1989). Educational requirements for certification. CPHCNP Newsletter 12(1):5-6.
31. Beecroft, P.C. & Papenhausen, J.L. (1989). Certification for specialty practice? Clinical Nurse Specialist 3(4):161.
32. Styles, M.M. (1989). On Specialization in Nursing: Toward a New Empowerment. Kansas City, MO: American Nurses Foundation.
33. Pearson, L.J. (1993). op. cit.
34. Study of Credentialing Launched. (1976). American Journal of Nursing 76:1893, 1895.
35. The Study of Credentialing in Nursing: A New Approach. (1979). Kansas City, MO: American Nurses' Association.
36. Credentialing in nursing: A new approach. (1979). Report of the Committee for the Study of Credentialing in Nursing. American Journal of Nursing 79:674-683.

37. NLN Accreditation Update (Report No. 3). (1980). New York: National League for Nursing. p. 1.
38. COAR. (1989). The Report of the Commission. Kansas City, MO: American Nurses Association.
39. Credentialing Health Manpower. (1977). Hyattsville, MO: U.S. Department of Health, Education, and Welfare.
40. NAACOG Certification Corporation. (July 1982). Newsletter. Special edition.
41. The Evolution of Nursing Professional Organizations. (1987). Kansas City, MO: American Academy of Nursing.
42. The NPDB sums up months of malpractice experience. (1992). American Journal of Nursing 92:9.
43. Moniz, D.M. (1992). The legal danger of written protocols and standards of practice. Nurse Practitioner 17(9):58-60.
44. Koniak-Griffin, D. (1987). Challenges for the clinical nurse specialist in the legal arena. Clinical Nurse Specialist 1(3):142-147.
45. Moss, K.F. (1985). California supreme court defines standard of care for NPs. The Nurse Practitioner 10(5):39-40, 42.
46. Trandel-Korenchuk, D.M. & Trandel-Korenchuk, K.M. (1979). Nursing malpractice insurance: A review of one policy. The Nurse Practitioner 4:11, 13, 15, 16-17, 19.
47. Professional Liability Series. (1987). Washington, DC: NAACOG.
48. Crane, M. (1979). Professional liability insurance: Occurrence versus claims-made policies. Newsletter of the Council of Primary Health Care Nurse Practitioners 2:6.
49. Brooke, P.S. (1989). The legal side: Shopping for liability insurance. American Journal of Nursing 89(2):171-172.
50. Northrup, C.E. (1980). Responding to the malpractice crisis. American Journal of Nursing 80:2245-2246.
51. Pearson, L.J. (1987). Comprehensive actuarial data on nurse practitioners . . . at long last. The Nurse Practitioner 12(12):6, 9-10.
52. Pearson, L.J. (1987). The liability insurance crisis. The Nurse Practitioner 12(6):8-10.
53. Senator Inouye introduces bill to set up no-fault federal malpractice system. (1978). American Journal of Nursing 78:187, 208.
54. Klein, C.A. (1986). Scope of practice. The Nurse Practitioner 11(11):67, 71-72.

7
Continuous Quality Improvement

Introduction

With the passage of the Professional Standards Review Organization bill (PSRO-P.L.92-603) in 1972 and the increased involvement of third party payers in monitoring the costs and quality of care, all health care providers have to concern themselves with some sort of evaluation and review system. The public is becoming increasingly vociferous in demanding accountability (1).

Clients, employers, and eventually third parties will demand that nurses be accountable for the cost and quality of the services they provide. Quality improvement represents a mechanism for accountability. In addition, a continuous quality improvement program can be structured to provide us with data to strengthen our case for third party reimbursement, to demonstrate the unique contribution nurses can make to quality health care, and to document our acceptance by clients (1a, 1b).

Continuous Quality Improvement: Some Definitions and Components

The focal point of health care quality has been quality assurance. This notion of quality has expanded beyond the concepts of measuring, monitoring, and evaluation to include the manager's responsibility and initiatives for system quality (Total Quality Management). The key aspects of TQM, stemming from the works of Juran and Deming, are client-orientation, commitment to quality by all levels and types of staff, organizational support and continuous improvement of the system as evidenced by prevention of problems and systematic, creative problem solving (3). Continuous quality improvement transcends the notion of QA as periodic evaluation of performance, as a reflection of quality, to become an integral part of the organization's vision which is operationalized in all facets of care delivery (3).

Attempts to define quality show the complexity of the concept. Any definition will reflect the biases of its author. At the same time, it is apparent that a quality improvement program must achieve at least a working agreement as to the quality of nursing care desired and must list the criteria that represent quality. One of the most useful definitions in the nursing literature states that quality of care is the observable characteristics that depict a desired and valued degree of excellence and its expected and observed variation (2).

Quality improvement programs are directed toward assuring some degree of excellence as defined by those responsible for the program and toward assuring accountability by health care providers for the quality of care they provide. An assumption in quality improvement is that every process can be improved. Juran (4) defines QI as "The organized creation of beneficial change... the attainment of unprecedented levels of performance."

The consumer should be the individual for whom we are assuring quality and to whom we are accountable. There are many, however, who would take issue with the consumer's rights or even ability to judge quality of care. Peers, institutions, and agencies as well as credentialing, licensing, and accrediting bodies now usurp this prerogative (5).

Strategies to assure quality are many and varied. We have become familiar with words like peer review, audit, and chart or record review. It is possible to incorporate a number of these strategies into the quality improvement process.

Quality improvement programs have addressed one or more of three domains: structure, process, and outcome. Structure evaluation involves looking at how the setting, the conditions, and the environmental factors affect the quality of care. Process evaluation examines the activities and behaviors of the nurse. Outcome measures demonstrate changes in the behaviors and attitudes of the clients.

The last component of quality improvement consists of the norms, criteria, and standards used as measures in the evaluation process (5).

Incorporating the questions of what we are assuring, for whom, how, the domains of structure, process, and outcome, and the variables we will choose to investigate, Schmadl (5) has come up with a definition which seems applicable within the context of advanced nursing practice. This definition assures the consumer a degree of excellence through an ongoing process of measuring and evaluating the setting and conditions of care, the process of nursing intervention, and/or client outcomes. It is predicated on using the pre-established criteria and standards. There is no end point to this quality improvement process. Evaluations lead to changes aimed at improving care, and the circle begins again (5).

Instituting a Quality Improvement Program in Advanced Practice

Defining Quality or Excellence

The first step in initiating a program for evaluating care is to define what is meant by excellence for the particular agency, program, or practice. It is helpful to review the objectives of the program, if they exist, and to decide if excellence is synonymous with achieving them. Usually, the objectives of an organization or a practice are broad enough to achieve consensus among those who will be involved in the quality improvement process. If the agency is a nonprofit, voluntary entity or a community or neighborhood center, there is a good chance that consumers have had input in formulating the objectives. Nurses in independent practice usually predicate their practice on goals related to the benefits they envision their services providing for clients. Some practices are based on community assessment, which yields data on the needs of the target population, and services are directed toward meeting those needs.

The first step in the quality improvement process affords the nurses involved an opportunity to discuss what they perceive as excellence for their practice, which can evolve into a clarification of values. It can help nurses understand where each is coming from and open up communication as differences are revealed. The hazard exists, of course, that being honest about one's values can have the effect of isolating one or more individuals from the group or creating two camps. Chances are, however, that members of the group are aware of differences already. The benefits to be gained through an honest discussion usually outweigh the hazards, particularly when an atmosphere is created that is nonthreatening and uncensoring of any opinion.

Quality Improvement — for Whom?

Once an agreement is reached as to the definition of excellence in practice, it is important to discuss for whose benefit the quality improvement program is being launched. If it is to satisfy the requirements for accreditation, licensure, credentialing, or third party regulations imposed by an official body or agency, then the methods chosen and the domains included should be those most appropriate for that task. Since a health care delivery system must address the needs of its clients, quality improvement would also necessarily be concerned with assuring a good quality of care for those persons. A quality improvement program might have as its sold purpose accountability to clients, or it might address the agency needs for accountability to accrediting and professional bodies as well.

Structure, Process or Outcome

The next step in establishing a program for quality improvement is to decide on which of the three domains -- structure, process, or outcome — to utilize for the process. Programs which look at structure might

examine components of services such as the setting and the conditions. Some of these components are listed in Table 7.1.
The decision as to which domain(s) to include will depend upon the purpose of, and target for, the quality improvement program. Criteria from licensing or accrediting bodies may dictate the domain. If the focus is on quality improvement for clients and total system quality, all three domains may be relevant. Certainly we as providers are concerned about the structure and process as well as outcomes and client satisfaction in all three domains.

Criteria, Standards, Norms

Criteria. Once the decision has been made as to the domains to include, the measurement (norms and/or standards) criteria must be set or chosen. A number of examples exist in the literature for criteria, norms, and standards for structure, process, and outcome. It is important to distinguish among these three as variables that might be chosen for examination. According to Bloch (6), a criterion is value free and is the name of a variable either believed or known to be a relevant indicator of the quality of client care. Criteria may be explicit statements of performance, circumstances, behavior or clinical status (7). Examples of criteria are included in many publications (7, 8, 9, 10, 11). Table 7.2 gives examples of structure, process, and outcome criteria for primary care.

Developing criteria for quality improvement programs is a very difficult task. Information must be obtained, and it is not always possible to find the kind of information from the literature that is valid and useful for a quality improvement program (12). For example, although one may wish to access information on management strategies and outcome criteria for hypertension control in adults sixty years and older, these data may be difficult to unearth. An extensive review of studies to date may be useful (13).

Establishing reliable criteria includes the following steps: literature search, examining the criteria that already exist; using experience and clinical expertise of those preparing criteria; and a good deal of thinking. Criteria should be based on a nursing model for practice (14).

Table 7.1. Measurement Domains for Quality Improvement*

STRUCTURE
Philosophy and objectives of agency, program, practice, institution
Organizational characteristics
Impact on quality of care
Resources
   fiscal
   equipment
   physical facilities
   personnel
Legal aspects to support mission
Management structure
Licensure, certification, accreditation status, approval, third-party regulations
Employees
   qualifications
   goals
   characteristics
   degree of colleagueship
   attitudes and values
   amount and kind of supervision available
Clients
   expectations
   attitudes
Value
   biophysical and psycho/cultural/social characteristics on entering system

PROCESS
Delivery of nursing care
   type
   behaviors of nurse
   sequence of events
   activities

(continued)

Table 7.1. (Continued)

   degree of skill of providers
Interactions
   among providers
   with clients
   with significant others
   inclusion of client, significant others
Techniques, procedures
Coordination of care
   among different components of the system
   among members of team
   continuity of care
Components of care
   among different components of the system
   among members of team
   continuity of care
Components of system
   utilization
   those available

OUTCOME
End results of nursing care
   change in health status
   client compliance and satisfaction
   change in client behavior, knowledge of mastery
   mortality
   morbidity
   disability
   social functioning
   activities of daily living

---

* Adapted from Schmadl, 1979, p. 463 (5); Bailit et al., 1975, pp. 155-158 (1); American Nurses Association. (1096). Quality Assurance Workbook, pp. 12-17. Kansas City, MO: American Nurses Association.

Table 7.2. Examples of Criteria in the Three Domains

STRUCTURE
National certification is required for each nurse in advanced practice.
The nurse practicing as a primary care provider must be a graduate of an approved certificate or master's program.
The caseload ratio is one nurse for every 350 clients.
Each professional provider is granted a minimum of five days per year for continuing studies.
Peer evaluation within the setting is intra- and interdisciplinary.
All members of the team have an equal voice in decision making for the agency.

PROCESS
The name and action of the drug will be explained to the client each time a prescription is written.
Assessment methods will be chosen on the basis of risk factors and client perception of the problem.
Significant others are included in the caregiving process.
All client assessments, planning, interventions, and evaluations are recorded using problem oriented format.
A problem list is to be prepared for each client at the first visit and updated at each subsequent visit.
A minimum of one-half hour will be allowed for each nurse visit and one hour for a first visit assessment.

OUTCOME
The annual rate of hospitalization is reduced in the target population.
Hypertension control as measured by mean blood pressure readings is attained.
Over one year a weight loss pattern will be established for obese clients.
Maintenance of optimal level of wellness for all clients in caseload as demonstrated by ability to perform activities of daily living at or above level of first visit.

Once criteria are developed, a panel of experts can be consulted as to their appropriateness for the concepts being measured. Establishing the validity of the criteria is another step in the process. To do this, multiple measures of the same concepts using external criteria can be done (15). Instruments for measuring criteria can be developed. Some examples of this exist in the literature (16), including the Ralph K. Davies Medical Center Nursing Care Planning System, Problems and Goals (17), and the Wisconsin System (18). A number of measures of quality of care that have been developed for nursing appear in the literature (13, 19).

Standards. Standards may be defined as achievable levels or ranges of performance which correspond with a criterion against which an actual performance may be compared (5). A standard may also be defined as compliance plus or minus a percentage of variance from a norm that is agreed upon as safe or excellent practice (20). A standard may also refer to a level of magnitude on a scale in order to make a statement about the quality of outcomes (21).

The American Nurses Association's standards for nursing practice are examples of standards of excellence for nursing practice that can be adopted or adapted for a practice, agency, or institution. A guide for implementing standards has also been prepared (22). The ANA standards pertinent to advanced practice are listed in this chapter's Bibliography. Other organizations such as the Association of Women's Health, Obstetric, and Neonatal Nurses (formerly NAACOG) have also developed standards and some of these appear in the Bibliography as well as the References (23).

Norms. A norm is a range or level of performance. It is generally the current "one" unless otherwise stated, and is generated from a descriptive investigation of a particular population, region, community, or group (6). Another definition of a norm describes it as a prevailing pattern or percentage of compliance (20). Norms may be statistical measures that are generated from a large data pool (21).

Mechanisms

Finally, methods must be chosen for the process of quality improvement. Audits, peer reviews, chart reviews, postcare client interviews or questionnaires, and staff conferences are some of the mechanisms that are employed (24). Methods for concurrent evaluation include open chart audits, client interviews and observations, interviewing and/or observing staff, and conferences of caregivers (25). Each of these methods might be appropriate for the nurse practitioner or clinical nurse specialist. Examples of ways to implement each of these mechanisms can be found in Table 7.3.

Audit. "Audit" is an umbrella term to mean the process of judging, retrospectively, the quality of nursing care with reference to professional standards. The audit has come to be synonymous with a retrospective chart review, the method generally used to obtain information on the "achievement, trends, and problems" for those under care (26). The audit gathers data on the client and setting, and a random sample of client records is chosen for review. A quality score is given along with remarks by the reviewer focusing on policy, procedures, and practices (27).

Outcome criteria can be used in the audit process (21). In ambulatory care with a long-term caseload, a retrospective audit might be done on a random sample of clients at the end of one year. Outcome criteria in relation to factors such as hypertension control, fertility control, weight loss or gain, and maintenance or restoration of the ability to perform activities of daily living might be evaluated as part of the audit. Audits can also use the standards of care prepared by professional organizations as criteria. Phaneuf (26) also suggests using Lesnik and Anderson's 7 functions of nursing: application and execution of physician's legal orders; observations of signs, symptoms and reactions; supervision of client; supervision of those who participate in care (except physicians); reporting and recording; application and execution of nursing procedures and techniques; and promotion of physical and emotional health through direction and teaching (28). Some of these are applicable to the advanced practice of nurses; others are not, or would

Table 7.3 Mechanisms for Quality Improvement in Nursing Care Settings

Mechanisms	Examples
Chart audit and review	Retrospective: pull charts randomly from file of clients not seen in last 6 months and identify strengths and deficits of care based on documentation in records.
	Open Chart: review of chart against predetermined criteria and feedback to caregiver.
	Group Audit: intra- or interdisciplinary, of randomly selected charts representing clients cared for by one or more members; review again predetermined criteria and critique of care.
	Independent Solo Practice: - Review of records with peer or peers consulting on a regular basis.
Patient interview and inspection	Specific interview and assessment as part of care process. Elicit subjective and objective data on patient perception of structure and process as well as outcome.
Postcare questionnaires	Instruments designed to elicit perceptions of structures, process, and/or outcome from clients' perceptions. May be filled out after a visit with a caregiver or at the end of a given time a client is in a particular practice or agency.
Utilization of instruments for measuring specific variables	Client assessment guides. Problem lists with outcome criteria and scoring system for these.
Staff interview or observation	Peer or interdisciplinary observation of the interview interactional process between provider and client; feedback after visit is over.

(continued)

Table 7.3 (continued)

Mechanisms	Examples
Group conferencing - concurrent	Inter- or intradisciplinary case review of selected clients; may also involve client, family, significant others. Focus may be on any or all of the three domains.
Postcare conferencing	Review of selected client cases no longer in caseload; involve all members of team who participated in care.
Postcare client interviews	Interview clients or group of clients after discharge from care system. In ambulatory setting, could be after a crisis and crisis resolution.

need modification. An example of an audit tool for nursing appears in Table 7.4.

In one example of audit for an ambulatory unit, charts for 25 clients who had visited an obstetric clinic over the past 12 months were randomly selected. Data were retrieved and then all staff participated in the review. The audit was carried out following methods developed by the Medical Quality Assurance Committee of the Joint Commission on Hospital Accreditation — the Performance Evaluation Procedure for Auditing and Improving Patient Care (PEP) (29).

Another example of the use of audit comes from a public health nursing agency. This agency used as criteria seven nursing functions and made judgments on a five-point scale from "Excellent" to "Unsafe" for each case audited through record review. The cases were clustered as to primary medical diagnoses (30). The results were then communicated by the nursing audit committee through supervisors to the staff nurses. The audit was considered to be one tool to appraise the quality of services (30).

Thus, the audit can be one mechanism used for a quality improvement program. As a method, it has both advantages and limitations. A

Table 7.4. Example of Audit Tool for Nursing Setting*

Client's name: _____
Client's sex: _____ Age: _____ Date of last Visit: _____
Number of visits in past 12 months: _____
Nursing diagnosis: _____

Hazardous events (biophysical and psychosocial)
  situational: _____
  developmental: _____
Hospitalizations in past 12 months: _____
Nursing visits signed and identified: _____
Problem list completed and updated to last visit: _____
Audit Criteria:

*Adapted from Phaneuf, 1976, Appendix 3 (26); Dorsey and Hussa, 1979, (29) pp. 41-43.

retrospective record audit assesses the quality of the record rather than of the care given. Setting criteria and standards is a difficult task. Rating scales are difficult to construct and by their very nature impose value judgments. Words which may be chosen, such as "good," "excellent," and "poor," have value-laden connotations.

Quality of nursing care is one facet of an interactional process involving client, perhaps family and/or significant others, and at times the community and other health care providers. Validity is dependent upon professional judgments. Reliability of judgments can be tested by experts in practice. Some of the knotty problems of using audit include who should do it and to what end. Although intended to be educational and constructive, audit may end up being used for purposes that tend to be punitive and destructive. Once the results of audit are ready, they must be used to improve care or the purpose of the process is lost. If change is short-lived, has the audit lost its purpose? How effective are attempts to effect change in professional behavior? The costs of the audit also must be considered. Are the ends worth the means? Is it a cost effective process? Does it achieve its purpose? (31).

The value of the audit to nurses can be multidimensional. It can bring about change in awareness, in perceptions of care, in knowledge, and in abilities. It can also serve as a consciousness-raising experience. If nurses have input into the process of developing criteria, factual knowledge can accrue. Audits also help to emphasize the role of nursing in client care and the independent nursing diagnoses and management strategies that are possible. The results of client teaching become apparent through the evaluation process.

Since a search of the literature is necessary for developing criteria, staff are exposed to and can have an opportunity to discuss current research and practices. The audit process can also generate research as a spin-off. Queries that arise as to definitions of nursing practice or the validity of management strategies can generate research questions.

Feedback affords nurses the opportunity to consider goals for client care and to evaluate reasons for failure to document care. An audit also reinforces the need for accountability through documentation. What has the potential of being a threatening process can be turned into a positive learning opportunity (32).

Peer Review. Peer review is the process by which a group of nursing colleagues evaluates the effectiveness of the work of its peers. Prior to implementing the process, criteria for the evaluation are developed. Criteria are then applied to an actual client care situation (33).

The American Nurses Association, in 1974, issued *Guidelines for Peer Review* through its Congress for Nursing Practice. Peer review has also been suggested as an integral part of developing the roles of advanced nurses (34). Peer review may also be interdisciplinary, as among members of a health care team such as might exist in a neighborhood health center or in outpatient clinics. For the nurse working in solo practice, peer review can be arranged through consultation with advanced practitioners working in similar settings.

Peer review can be ongoing or periodic. It can be based on the standards of care and the scope of practice developed through professional organizations or upon criteria established for a particular practice or agency (35).

Peer review can be conducted in a number of different ways. One of these is chart audit and review. Another is through direct observation of a client care episode followed by an evaluation. The nurse being reviewed may present a client case or selected clients from her/his caseload for review.

Peer review for advanced nurses can include evaluation of nurse developed protocols, knowledge and management strategies, incorporation of education, philosophy of practice, and client feedback. Forms can be developed for the review process and used for evaluating and sharing sessions and as a guide for improving care (33). An example of a peer review form can be found in Table 7.5. Another example is described and evaluated in the work of Goodwin, Jacox, Prescott and colleagues (38, 39, 40).

As with any evaluation process, there are both advantages and some pitfalls. There are satisfactions to be gained from documenting the health care nurses are providing. Nurses also can gain an awareness of the importance of developing instruments to measure components of health care. Quality of care can be improved. For nurses working in isolated areas or in solo practice, peer review provides a mechanism for sharing knowledge and experience (37.) Peer review is one method for implementing standards of practice and for controlling practice within the profession (41). Peer review encourages examination of self and one's own practice. It can serve to encourage self-study and continuing education. Levels of competence are identified (36).

Peer review has some pitfalls as well. It can be anxiety-producing and threatening. There is a temptation to engage in "in-group self-protection at the expense of the public (41). There is also a danger that interests in economic welfare will usurp interests in quality and cost of care (41). Peer review cannot be forced on any nurse. It will not be effective if the nurse does not see it as her/his responsibility and right (42). Time and distance can be inhibiting factors, especially in rural areas (37).

Table 7.5 Peer Review Worksheet

Nurse:_____ Reviewer:_____
Setting:_____ Date of review:_____
A. Protocols (developed by nurse)
   Literature
   Type
   Appropriateness of management strategies
   Evaluation tool
B. Colleague interaction
   Use of referrals
   Collaboration with other nurses - peer consultation
   Collaboration and coordination with other providers
   Chart review and results
C. Nurse knowledge and preparation
   Continuing education: when, what?
   Journals read regularly
   Examples of knowledge of current research and application in practice
   Engaged in research at present? If so, what?
   Record keeping
      Complete?
      POMR
      Reflective of appropriate management strategies
      Patient education - documentation
D. Observations
   Interactions: appropriate, quality
   Nursing process
   Client assessment, planning, intervention, evaluation
   Charting reflective of process
   Plans for follow-up
   Measure of client satisfaction with care
E. Nurse's philosophy: ability to articulate; familiarity with scope of practice, standards of care; model for practice

Comments of nurse:
Comments of reviewer:
Plans based on assessment:

Interviews and Questionnaires. These can be used to elicit input as to clients' perceptions of care. Interviewing is more flexible and has a higher response rate than questionnaires, although it is a more expensive method. Also, responses may reflect the client's attempts to please the interviewer (43).

Questionnaires can assure confidentiality and are less costly and time-consuming than interviews. They are especially useful when geographic distribution is great. They can be handed out at the end of a visit or mailed to a sample of clients. However, the response rate is usually low, items may be skipped, and there is usually no opportunity to elicit further information. The respondents' level of understanding and language must be taken into account (43). The use of a computer should be considered when constructing the instrument. An example of an evaluation questionnaire appears in Table 7.6.

Client feedback is important, if not critical, to the health care delivery process. Input reflects the opinions of consumers and can thus help nurses improve public relations, foster morale among providers, and dispel tensions between consumers and providers (44). Feedback to the client following the evaluation will help to facilitate communication and encourage openness.

Some agencies also hold an open group meeting periodically for the purposes of review and evaluation. Clients can then meet with members of the caregiving team (44). This could be done both for individual clients and for a group.

Summary

Quality improvement is an important component of the caregiving process. Accountability to consumers is increasing in importance as demands are voiced and is already, in some cases, tied to third-party reimbursement for services. Several tasks remain in the ongoing process of developing models for improvement programs for nursing. We need to continue to develop outcome criteria for clients. At the same time, nursing needs to develop outcome criteria for clients. At the same time, nursing needs to develop nursing care and management-specific

Table 7.6 Client Questionnaire

In order to improve our services, we would appreciate your taking a few minutes to answer the following questions.

1. When you came to the clinic, were you generally well-received and treated courteously by the staff?
   Yes ____ No ____

2. Once at the clinic, how long did you wait to be seen?
   Less than 15 minutes ____ 15-30 minutes ____
   30-60 minutes ____ Over an hour ____

3. How would you rate the competence of the nurse who saw you in meeting your needs?
   Outstanding ____ Above average ____ Average ____
   Below average ____ Way below average ____

4. How would you rate the explanation of examination procedures and care you received?
   Outstanding ____ Above average ____ Average ____
   Below average ____ Way below average ____

5. How would you rate the concern of the nurse with your feelings as a person?
   Outstanding ____ Above average ____ Average ____
   Below average ____ Way below average ____

6. Do you think such concern is appropriate as part of care?
   Always ____ Almost always ____ Sometimes ____
   Rarely ____ Never ____

7. Did your problem require consultation with a physician?
   Yes ____ No ____

8. If not, did you wish to see a physician?
   Yes ____ No ____

(continued)

Table 7.6 (continued)

9. Prior to this visit, how many times have you had a health exam as an adult?
   Never ____ Once ____ More than once ____

10. If you answered "Once" or "More than once" to Question 9, where was the exam (exams) performed?
    Physician's office or clinic ____
    This clinic ____ Other nurse's office or clinic ____

11. If you have been to other health care services clinics, how would you compare care in this clinic with those other clinics?
    Much better ____ Better ____ Equal to ____
    Worse ____ Much worse ____

12. In the future, if you have similar health care needs, would you prefer to see:
    An advanced practice nurse ____ A physician ____
    Doesn't matter ____

13. Please add any suggestions or comments concerning health care.

Thank you! Your cooperation will help us to serve you better.

---

outcome criteria. Bloch (45) has suggested establishing a national clearinghouse on nursing evaluation to foster coordination and the sharing of ideas and to avoid duplication of work. This center could also establish a list of experts and consultants.

Advanced practitioners must take the lead in redefining the system that rewards nurses for professional excellence in quality improvement in patient care. Advanced practitioners must incorporate QI principles and tools in daily practice. "Our time has come: CQI is a breakthrough where nurses can demonstrate a major positive impact on quality health care delivery in the 1990's" (46).

REFERENCES

1. Bailit, H., Lewis, J., Hochheiser, L., & Bush, N. (1975). Assessing the quality of care. Nursing Outlook 23:153-159.
1a. Malone, B.L. (1986). Evaluation of the clinical nurse specialist. American Journal of Nursing 86:1375-1377.
1b. Ingersoll, G.L. (1988). Evaluating the impact of a clinical nurse specialist. Clinical Nurse Specialist 2(3):150-155.
2. Zimmer, M.J. (1974). Quality assurance for outcomes of patient care. Nursing Clinics of North America 9:305-315.
3. Kirk, R. (1992). The big picture: Total quality management and continuous quality improvements. Journal of Nursing Administration 22:24-31.
4. Juran, J.M. (1989). Juran on Leadership for Quality: An Executive Handbook. New York: The Free Press, p. 28.
5. Schmadl, J.C. (1979). Quality assurance: Examination of the concept. Nursing Outlook 27:462-465.
6. Bloch, D. (1977). Criteria, standards, norms - crucial terms in quality assurance. Journal of Nursing Administration 1:22, 26.
7. Mayers, M.G., Norby, R.B., & Watson, A.B. (1977). Quality Assurance for Patient Care. New York: Appleton-Century-Crofts, p. 21.
8. Nicholls, M.E. (1977). Terminology in quality assurance. In: M.E. Nicholls & V.G. Wessels (Eds.) Nursing Standards and Nursing Process. Wakefield, MA: Contemporary Publishing.
9. Levitt, M.K., Stern, N.B., Becker, K.L., Zaiken, H., Hangasky, S. & Wilcox, P.M. (1985). A performance appraisal tool for nurse practitioners. The Nurse Practitioner 10(8):28-29, 33.
10. Fenton, M.V. (1985). Identifying competencies of clinical nurse specialists. Journal of Nursing Administration 15(12):31-37.
11. Steele, S. & Fenton, M.V. (1988). Expert practice of clinical nurse specialists. Clinical Nurse Specialist 2:45-52.

12. Williamson, J.W. (1980). Information management in quality assurance. Nursing Research 29:78-81.
13. Lang, N.M. & Clinton, J.F. (1984). Assessment of quality of nursing care. In: H.H. Werley & J.J. Fitzpatrick (Eds.) Annual Review of Nursing Research (vol. 2). New York: Springer Publishing Company. pp. 135-163.
14. Runtz, S.F. & Urtel, J.G. (1983). Evaluating your practice via a nursing model. Nurse Practitioner 8:30, 32, 37-40.
15. Horn, B.J. (1980). Establishing valid and reliable criteria: A researcher's perspective. Nursing Research 29:88-90.
16. Nicholls, M.E. & Wessells, V.G. (Eds.) (1977). Nursing Standards and Nursing Process. Wakefield, MA: Contemporary Publishing. p. 33.
17. Howe, M.J. (1980). Developing instruments for measurement of criteria: A clinical nursing practice perspective. Nursing Research 29:100-103.
18. Hover, J. & Zimmer, M.J. (1978). Nursing quality assurance: The Wisconsin System. Nursing Outlook 26: 242-248.
19. Chance, K.S. (1980). The quest of quality: An exploration of attempts to define and measure quality nursing care. Image 12:41-45.
20. Mayers, M.G., Norby, R.B. & Watson, A.B. (1977). Quality Assurance for Patient Care. New York: Appleton-Century-Crofts. p. 29.
21. Zimmer, M.J. & Lang, N.M. (1976). Evaluation of patient health/wellness outcomes. In: M.C. Phaneuf (Ed.) The Nursing Audit (2nd ed.). New York: Appleton-Century-Crofts. pp. 161-168.
22. A Plan for Implementation of the Standards of Nursing Practice. (1977). Kansas City, MO: American Nurses' Association.
23. Standards for Nursing Care of Women and Newborns. 4th ed. (1991). Washington, DC: NAACOG.
24. Mayers, M.G., Norby, R.B., & Watson, A.B. (1977). Quality

Assurance for Patient Care. New York: Appleton-Century-Crofts. pp. 12-13.
25. Ibid., p. 14.
26. Phaneuf, M.C. (1976). The Nursing Audit (2nd ed.). New York: Appleton-Century-Crofts. p. 3.
27. Ibid., p. 35.
28. Lesnik, M.J. & Anderson, B.E. (1955). Nursing Practice and the Law. Philadelphia: J.B. Lippincott. pp. 259-260.
29. Dorsey, B. & Hussa, R.K. (1979). Evaluating ambulatory care: Three approaches. Journal of Nursing Administration 74:24-35.
30. Phaneuf, M.C. (1969). Quality of care: Problems of measurement. American Journal of Public Health 59:1829-1831.
31. Donabedian, A. (1969). Some issues in evaluating the quality of nursing care. American Journal of Public Health 59:1833-1836.
32. Moore, K.R. (1979). What nurses learn from nursing audit. Nursing Outlook 27:254-258.
33. Tobin, H.M., Yoder, P.S., Hull, P.K. & Scott, B.C. (1974). The Process of Staff Development: Components for Change. St. Louis: C.V. Mosby. p. 129.
34. Murray, B.L. (1972). A case for independent group nursing practice. Nursing Outlook 20:60-63.
35. Koltz, C.J. (1979). Private Practice in Nursing. Germantown, MD: Aspen. pp. 200-201.
36. Vengroski, S.M. & Saarmann, L. (1978). Peer review in quality assurance. American Journal of Nursing 78:2094-2096.
37. Hiserote, J.L., Bultemeier, K., Kimberly, S.L., Nicoll, J.C. & Wheeler, K. (1980). Peer review among rural clinics. The Nurse Practitioner 5:30-32.
38. Goodwin, L., Prescott, P., Jacox, A., & Collar, M. (1981). The nurse practitioner rating scale II. Nursing Research 30:270-276.
39. Prescott, P.A., Jacox, A., Collar, M. & Goodwin, L. (1981). The nurse practitioner rating form I. Nursing Research 30:223-228.
40. Jacox, A., Prescott, P., Collar, M. & Goodwin, L. (1981). A

Primary Care Process Measure. The Nurse Practitioner Rating Form. Wakefield, MA: Nursing Resources.
41. Ramphal, M. (1974). Peer review. American Journal of Nursing 74:63-67.
42. Hauser, M.A. (1975). Initiation into peer review. American Journal of Nursing 75:2204-2207.
43. Marriner, A. (1979). The research process in quality assurance. American Journal of Nursing 79:2158-2161.
44. Froebe, D.J. & Bain, R.J. (1976). Quality Assurance Programs and Controls in Nursing. St. Louis: C.V. Mosby. pp. 81-82.
45. Bloch, D. (1975). Evaluation of nursing care in terms of process and outcome: Issues in research and quality assurance. Nursing Research 24:256-263.
46. Koch, M.W. (1991). Continuous quality improvement implications for nursing administration. The Facilitator. Council on Nursing Administration, ANA: Kansas City, MO: 17:4-6.

BIBLIOGRAPHY

Aguayo, R. (1990). Dr. Deming. The American Who Taught the Japanese about Quality. New York: Carol Publishing Group.

Arikan, V.L. (1991). Total quality management: Applications to nursing service. Journal of Nursing Administration 21:46-50.

Casalou, R. (1991). Total quality management in health care. Hospitals & Health Services Administration 36:134-146.

Deming, W.E. (1986). Out of the Crisis. Cambridge, MA: Institute of Technology Center for Advanced Engineering Study

Gillem, T.R. (1988). Deming's 14 points and hospital quality: Responding to the consumer's demand for the best value in health care. Nursing Quality Assurance 2:70-80.

Gitlow, H. & Gitlow, S. (1987). The Deming Guide to Quality and Competitive Position. Englewood, NJ: Prentice-Hall.

Houston, S. & Luquire, R. (1991). Measuring success: CNS perfor mance appraisal. Clinical Nurse Specialist 5(4):204-209.
Howard, J. & Wolff, P. (1992). Evaluation of clinical nurse specialist practice. Clinical Nurse Specialist 6(1):28-35.
Kearnes, D.R. (1992). A productivity tool to evaluate NP practice: Monitoring clinical time spent in reimbursable patient-related activities. The Nurse Practitioner 17(4):50; 52; 55.
Kirk, R. & Hoesing, H. (1991). Common Sense Quality Management: The Nurse's Guide. West Dundee, IL: S/N Publications.
Leming, T. (1991). Quality customer service: Nursing's new challenge. Nursing Administration Quarterly 15:6-12.
Martin, J.P. (1989). From implication to reality through a unit-based quality assurance program. Clinical Nurse Specialist 3(4):192-196.
Naylor, M.D., Munro, B.H. & Brooten, D.A. (1991). Measuring the effectiveness of nursing practice. Clinical Nurse Specialist 5(4):210-215.
Peer Review Guidelines, 1988*
Peglow, D.M., Klatt-Ellis, T., Stelton, S., Cutillo-Schmitter, T., Howard, J. & Wolff, P. (1992). Evaluation of clinical nurse specialist practice. Clinical Nurse Specialist 6(1):28-35.
Waltz, C.F. & Sylvia, B.M. (1991). Accountability and outcome measurement: Where do we go from here? Clinical Nurse Specialist 5(4):202-203.

STANDARDS:

Nursing Standards for Early Intervention Services for Children and Families at Risk. California Nurses Association, 1990.
Standards and Scope of Hospice Nursing Practice, 1987.*
Standards and Scope of Gerontological Nursing Practice, 1987.*
Standards for Care of Women and Newborns. 4th ed. Washington, DC: Nurses' Association of the American College of Obstetricians and Gynecologists, 1991.

Standards for the Clinical Nurse Specialist in Developmental Disabilities/Handicapping Conditions. Nursing Divisions: American Association of University Affiliated Programs and American Association on Mental Deficiency, 1987.
Standards for Organized Nursing Services and Responsibilities of Nurse Administrators Across All Settings, 1988.*
Standards for Professional Nursing Education, 1984.*
Standards of Addictions Nursing Practice with Selected Diagnoses and Criteria, 1987.*
Standards of Cardiovascular Nursing Practice, 1981.*
Standards of Child and Adolescent Psychiatric and Mental Health Nursing Practice, 1988.*
Standards of Clinical Nursing Practice, 1991.*
Standards of College Health Nursing Practice, 1986.*
Standards of Community Health Nursing Practice, 1986.*
Standards of Home Health Nursing Practice, 1986.*
Standards of Maternal-Child Health Nursing Practice, 1983.*
Standards of Medical-Surgical Nursing Practice, 1974.*
Standards of Nursing Practice in Correctional Facilities, 1985.*
Standards of Oncology Nursing Practice, 1987.*
Standards of Pediatric Oncology Nursing Practice, 1978.*
Standards of Practice for the Perinatal Nurse Specialist, 1985.*
Standards of Practice for the Primary Health Care Nurse Practitioner, 1987.*
Standards of Psychiatric and Mental Health Nursing, 1985.*
Standards for Psychiatric Consultation-Liaison Nursing Practice, 1992.
Standards of Rehabilitation Nursing Practice, 1986.*
Standards of School Nursing Practice, 1983.*

** Published by the American Nurses' Association, Kansas City, MO. (now of Washington, D.C.)

8

The Role of Research in Advanced Practice

Introduction

Research should be an integral part of the advanced practitioner's role, primarily for two reasons. First, if nursing is to continue to move toward a more influential position concerning health care policy and delivery, it will need to demonstrate competence in knowledge and action. To quote Gortner et al., "Research is the means by which much of that knowledge is accumulated, refined, and extended" (1). Second, if nurses are to justify their roles as providers within the health care delivery system, we are going to have to document that what they do for clients makes a difference. Escalating costs dictate the need for professional accountability. To be accountable, measurable outcomes are needed. Research is the means by which outcomes can be validated, the value of nursing management demonstrated, and the practice quantified as unique and, in some cases, superior to that of other health care professionals. Since we compete, in part, for a market of clients, we must be able to document what we have to offer them.

Since not all nurses have the skills to conduct research, levels of participation must necessarily vary. Participants in research can be subjects, research assistants, consultants on content and nursing aspects, or principal investigators for a project (2). In addition, all nurses in advanced practice can become knowledgeable consumers of research.

Historical Background

Prior to 1952, a total of 259 nursing articles can be identified as having a basis in research. Most of these dealt with issues of nursing function, welfare, curriculum, and procedures. Only a few clinical research articles appeared, mostly in the area of maternal-child health. Of the authors of these articles, only 60% were nurses (3). The inventory of nurses published by the ANA represented the first systematic attempt at data collection about the profession. Yet, as early as 1949, Esther Lucile Brown identified research as a component of the nursing role (4), and in 1950, the National League for Nursing Publication Conference emphasized the need for research to help students solve problems (5).

The first issue of *Nursing Research* was published in June 1952. That was also the year in which the Joint Committee on Nursing Research and Studies published its philosophy and Plan of Action (6). In the following year, the Institute of Research and Service in Nursing Education was established at Teachers College, Columbia University, and Virginia Henderson of Yale's School of Nursing and Leo Simmons, a member of Yale's Sociology Department, began a survey and assessment of nursing research (3). Such was the growth of the movement that at the 1960 ANA convention over 800 nurses attended the Research Conference Group (3).

In 1965, the first nursing conference dedicated to research was held under the joint sponsorship of the American Nurses Association and the American Nurses Foundation, the latter with origins dating to the 1950 ANA series of studies on the functions of nursing (3).

Early publications on nursing research include *Nursing Research: Survey and Assessment* by Simmons and Henderson, 1964 (7), *Fundamentals of Research in Nursing* by Fox, 1966 (8), and *Better Patient Care through Nursing Research* by Abdellah and Levine,

1965 (9).

The ANA convention in 1974 witnessed the presentation of two research papers to standing room only crowds. Of particular importance is that both papers focused on clinical nursing concerns and their relationship to research (5).

Thus, nursing research has, to quote Elizabeth Carnegie, "Come of age within the past 25 years" (10). The number of nurses prepared at the graduate level has grown from only a few in the late twenties to an estimated more than 112,000 in 1992 (11). Impetus has been added over the past three decades by the availability of federal nurse traineeship monies to support preparation of nurses at the master's and doctoral levels and availability of some federal monies to support nursing research projects.

Advanced Practice Research Today

Because of the importance of research to practice and to the role of the nurse in advanced practice, it is important for those without research skills to acquire them through continuing their formal education and through participation, at some level, in the research process.

Jacox and Norris have written that "the need for careful research designed to answer relevant questions is paramount for the nurse practitioner movement" (12). Nurses practice as primary care providers in settings unfamiliar to physicians, such as in homes and in geographic areas where there are no physicians. The populations they serve may be the poor, the aged, or minorities. Nurses focus on health care and on return to optimal level of functioning and not on curing illnesses, although they may be involved in illness care. They utilize management strategies that incorporate self-care, health education, and collaboration with clients. They assist clients to adapt to limitations. All of these facets of nursing practice in primary care roles need to be researched in order to strengthen the power base of nurses in advanced practice. We need also to explore health and illness behaviors and measure the outcomes of our nursing management on these as well as on pathological states (13).

Barnard (14) emphasizes the need for practitioners to collaborate in the entire research process. While Barnard uses the term practitioner in a broad sense, the message is certainly applicable to nurses engaged in advanced practice roles.

Research has a number of important contributions to make beyond affecting and enhancing the quality of care and promoting health. It provides an avenue for introducing innovations and change. It lends credibility to lobbying processes by providing data to support legislation on issues such as reimbursement for nursing management (12). Research can be used to identify communities of underserved clients and to document their health care needs.

Identifying Researchable Problems

The first step in the research process is to identify researchable problems for nursing (15, 16). While it is not within the scope of this book to teach the research process, it seems pertinent to single out this step within the context of advanced practice. (A number of research references appear in Appendix G.) The rapid growth of nursing's entry into primary care and case management has raised many important questions about advanced practice roles. Loretta Ford (17) has raised some important questions in creating her research agenda for primary care. She suggests a need to examine the impact of interventions by nurse practitioners on the health status of populations served. Research should also be directed toward examining the organizational changes that will be necessary to deliver the quality of care inherent in the nurse practitioner model.

Financing of care by nurses is also a critical issue, particularly in this time of spiralling costs within the health care delivery system. In the aftermath of the growth of clinical specialist programs since 1954 and of nurse practitioner programs since 1965, it is important to step back and examine the fit between these educational programs and the needs of society.

There is also a need to examine the interface between nurses prepared for advanced practice with other professionals, including nurses (17). Studies of the unique contributions nursing can make to client care and of the importance of nursing to health care delivery are needed. The quality of the experience a client has with a nurse in advanced practice may be an important variable in the client's choice of provider. Nurse practitioners and clinical nurse specialists must be able to demonstrate the benefits of their management if they expect to be reimbursed for it (18). Data are needed to hold nursing's own in the political arena and to support its positions in the development of public policy for health care provision (19).

Clinical nurses specialists increasingly are expected to incorporate research activities into their roles. Cronenwett has written a succinct and useful guide to fulfilling that expectation (20, 21). Collaboration between clinical nurse specialists and faculty members in nursing can be one way to fulfill this expectation and benefit both nursing practice and nursing education (22, 23, 24). A number of broad issues for research readily suggest themselves: the fit between educational preparation and role expectations; role development and role performance after completion of a master's program; characteristics of practice settings and client populations; and intervention and outcome studies with selected client groups.

Directions for research for nurse practitioners have also been identified. Early studies focused on characteristics of nurse practitioners. As the role has matured, researchers might turn their efforts toward prescriptive theory building (25).

Put another way, nurses in advanced practice need to research issues of role definition, their credibility as providers of care, the politics of health care delivery, and the ethical issues surrounding the delivery of care. The controversies concerning educational preparation for new roles and functions need to be explored. There is a need to define research for nursing practice; to address the ethical issues involved in human subject research; to inspect the progress of the state of the art in research within our profession; and to establish guidelines for educational preparation for nurse researchers (22).

Incorporating the Role of Researcher into Practice

One of the most critical issues in research for nurses in advanced roles is finding the time to do it. The many demands on a nurse's time often preclude research as an integral part of his or her practice. Research is pushed to the back burner and the someday that it will be undertaken never arrives. Conversely, a mentoring relationship can foster research. An institutional commitment to research as an integral part of the role of the clinical nurse specialist also helps to makes doing research possible (24a). Clinical nurse specialists also have a role to play in facilitating research (23).

The major impediment to incorporating research into the nursing role is the belief that research is somehow separate and magical. Yet each of us in our everyday practice collects reams of data. Collaborative projects with other providers may be possible utilizing these data. It is also sometimes feasible to combine research and demonstration programs. The initiation of a new format for delivering services or establishing a demonstration project can provide the impetus for research (27).

Developing and implementing a role (such as that of nurse practitioner or clinical specialist) within an agency can generate research questions. The daily statistical records on clients seen, the problems they present, and the management strategies used provide a wealth of data. The development, implementation, and evaluation of protocols for nursing management may be necessary for practice within a particular state of institution. The product of this process — outcomes for clients — could be the subject of a piece of nursing research.

Cluster studies might be possible within an agency, perhaps with collaboration between providers and faculty utilizing the agency for student experiences. Service agencies need to develop clinical research programs and to involve their staff in research (26). Several collaborative models have been developed and show promise for replication in other agencies and institutions (27, 28).

Funding for Research

Research can be costly if it involves materials, equipment, and time over and above those that are part of the service role of the individual or institution. Access to computer services for data retrieval, storage, analysis, and literature searches may also be necessary and will represent an expense if such services are not provided by the institution. Thus, soliciting support for research outside of the employing agency or, for the independent practitioner, outside of her or his own funds, may be necessary, and a grant may need to be applied for.

Resources to help you write a grant for funding are included in the bibliography of this chapter, and Appendices E and F at the end of the book list resources on grantsmanship and funding sources. Courses on grant writing are useful and so is eliciting help from someone who has written a successful grant.

Impediments to Research

In general, women have not been socialized into roles as thinkers, analyzers, and questioners. Additionally, women must often surmount difficulties not encountered by their male colleagues. The average working woman puts in 80 hours a week, the average man puts in 50 hours. Children and household responsibilities often are distractors. Women thus must be creative in order to be creative. The orderly nature of nursing can stifle creativity also, for nurses are educated to be neat and compliant, assets that may be impediments in the research process, according to Notter (26). Nurses are often trapped into believing that research must be quantitative and abstract, whereas action research (research which is incorporated into practice) may be more appropriate to the questions that must be answered to validate our practice. We need to continue to move away from the medical model and generate and utilize our own models for research (26). Nurses have been characterized as doers rather than thinkers and we need to divest ourselves of that image. We need to focus on defining nursing and nursing's role. More replication studies are needed to advance nursing science (26). We have depended too long upon the research generated through master's theses and doctoral dissertations (5)—we need more postdoctoral research and studies over time. Finally, we need to fully incorporate the role of researcher into our image of nursing. If we continue to view it as an awkward appendage, an honor reserved for a chosen few, or as an albatross hung around our necks by some zealous dean, department head, or nurse administrator, we will continue to view research as just one more demand on our time.

Incorporating Research Findings into Practice

"The translation of research is a responsibility of practitioners" (28a). Embracing research as an integral part of the role of the nurse in advanced practice means not only involvement in conducting research, but also being an intelligent consumer of the research generated by others. Barnard (28b) states that the key to this is "getting researchers and clinicians to interact." A survey of nurses in New York State disclosed that one of the obstacles to applying research findings was obtaining these findings. The most frequently read nursing journals are those that contain the smallest number of research studies, according to Miller and Messinger (29), and this is borne out by recent data indicating that the journal with the largest number of readers publishes few, if any, research studies.

Conferences, inservice programs, and the distribution of summaries of research findings were cited as other sources of information in addition to journal articles (29). Incorporating into basic nursing education programs the skills of reading and critiquing research intelligently will accelerate the utilization of research findings (5). So will the inclusion of a research component in programs designed to prepare nurses for advanced practice roles.

One model for disseminating research findings to staff nurses has evolved. This was a deliberate and systematic plan built into the research process to identify and reach a larger population of nurse practitioners, and was developed to expedite communication from researcher to practitioners. In this model, the findings were translated and evaluated (30). This represents one step forward in closing the gap between researchers and those in nursing who care directly for clients. Nurses in advanced practice can serve as facilitators for research utilization (31).

Exploring utilization of research among nurses in advanced practice is important to increasing their roles in facilitating utilization by others (32). A barrier to incorporating research findings into practice is nurses' self-image (33). Nurses do not always see themselves as capable of shaping their own practice. Exposure to research findings and evaluation of these findings for their implications for practice will encourage research use (34). Skills in using research are also necessary if research is to be applied to practice (35). The closer researchers and practitioners move together, the more relevant research will be to the problems practitioners encounter in their management of client care and the more likely that the results of nursing research will effect change in practice.

Publishing

If research findings are to be applied in practice, they must be widely disseminated to practitioners. Thus, the publication of management strategies, protocols, case studies, and other data generated through practice and research can contribute to the body of knowledge about health care as delivered by nurses.

Why publish? Styles (36) has written that "the primary reason to publish is because the future of the profession depends on it." The profession needs to have evidence of its scholarship through publication. Then, too, there is the personal thrill of seeing one's work in print, of being recognized as an author, and of receiving the professional rewards accorded to published authors (36).

The first hurdle to cross in writing for publication is fear. Each of us is tempted to wallow in the mire of fear of publishing. Our procrastination strategies would win prizes for the creativity they demonstrate. In desperation, we retreat to the old cliche, "Oh, I can't write." If you can talk, you can write, and as a nurse, chances are you do a lot of both as part of your everyday role.

Start small if you feel you won't have enough to say for an article or if the thought of 10 to 15 pages is overwhelming. Write a letter to the editor. Co-author your first writing effort (37). Both of these techniques help to overcome fear.

Another step in overcoming fear is to read. Critique the articles you read. Ask yourself, "Could I have written that?" "Could I have done better?" "Did the opening paragraph invite me to read further?"

Write about what you know. In preparing a manuscript for publication on a research project, think of your audience. They will want to know who, what, where, how, and why, and, most importantly, the implications of your article or book for their practice. Emphasize how you have incorporated the research process into your practice (if you have), cite related studies, and document accurately. It is frustrating to try to track down a reference that is incorrectly cited.

The steps in writing are similar to those in nursing process. First, assess your practice and your strengths as a nurse in advanced practice. Write about protocols or management strategies you have developed. If you have completed a research project, evaluate the outcomes for possible articles. What would you as an advanced practitioner most like to share from your experience or your research?

The arguments for or against selecting a refereed journal are many. A refereed journal is one which utilizes the opinions of three or more experts in the field who review a manuscript so that the journal's editor can decide whether to publish it. These are generally independent and blind reviews to eliminate bias. A list of the referee status of nursing journals is available (38). The value of the opinions of experts in the field is that the editor benefits from diverse points of view (39). The reviews also allow for a submitted article to be judged against the body of substantive knowledge specific to the discipline (40). Conversely, it can be argued that the review panel can turn into "The Establishment" (40). The debate has no clear solution (38). To select a refereed versus a non-refereed journal must remain an individual decision. Most important is selecting a journal which publishes articles of the type you wish to write.

Peruse journals in the field and select one which seems appropriate to the topic you have in mind. After selecting one, check it concerning article length, number of manuscript copies to submit, and other information pertinent to authors (41). This information is usually found on the page with the table of contents and publisher's information. You can also write to the editor and request information. A comparison of 92 journals was published in 1991 with respect to this type of information (38).

Plan your article. Research the topic or gather together the material from your study and organize it into subgroups. You may want to develop a detailed outline and work from that. It is useful to have on hand a number of reference works that will give you information on preparing your manuscript. A list of suggested references on or related to writing is included in this chapter's bibliography.

If you plan to include tables or graphs, lay them out so they can be typed or reproduced easily. Avoid the use of "alphabet soup" by spelling out all but the most obvious terms. Keep tables as brief and uncluttered as possible. Try to convey only the most important information and leave out unnecessary details and items peripheral to the main ideas or findings. Photographs should be clear, glossy, and black and white and in only enough detail to convey your message. Photos are expensive to reproduce, so use only those essential to the message of your article. Line drawings (not shaded), on the other hand, involve no extra printing expense. Often journals will assist you by providing photographs or line drawings if they will enhance the article. Sources of photographs run the gamut from those you or your friends or colleagues take, to professional medical photographers, to archives. The Bettmann Archive in New York City is one source of historical photographs available for a relatively nominal fee. A computer makes sophisticated graphics possible.

A writer's workshop can be helpful, particularly for the beginner. A workshop is generally designed to assist those who are novices as nurse authors to develop their ideas and carry them through to the point of submission to a journal. The format is usually informal and involves the active participation of those attending. Group support is a side benefit. Within the security of a peer group, a workshop can also help prepare the potential writer with some of the basic ingredients: how to write a query letter or an outline, and how to overcome some of the first-time jitters about the review process.

In the end, however, "a workshop is no substitute for writing and writing, and *writing*" (43). Making time to write is important. Some helpful hints for advanced practice nurses appeared in a professional newsletter (44). If you need a block of time, set it aside and use it only for writing. Since time will not make itself, you will have to make the time to write.

Finally, when there is no way out, sit down and write. Don't worry about writing in sequence from beginning to end. If the introduction just won't come, begin to write with the part that seems easiest. Set short-term goals and reward yourself when goals are attained. Write in a straightforward manner and use the active voice whenever possible. Avoid sounding pedantic or pompous. Double-check all figures, totals, and tables, and use up-to date information (42). Most of all, keep writing.

An evaluation of the product of your efforts can take several forms. Solicit peer review. Ask your colleagues to read what you have written and invite them to offer suggestions. If what you have written is clear to them, then you have made your points well. If questions arise when they read your manuscript, incorporate the answers in your rewrite. If grammar is not your strong point, use one of the standard guide or style manuals and seek out a reviewer who has skills in English. Set your manuscript aside for a few days after you complete the first draft, then go back and reread it and see if it says what you mean to convey.

Follow your potential publisher's specifications for typing, style of documentation, margins, and so on precisely. A well-organized, neat manuscript makes a favorable impression regardless of content. If you do not type well, have someone type the manuscript for you. Preparation of a manuscript on a word processor is ideal. Proofread and correct carefully. Send the manuscript with the requested number of copies and include any supplementary material specified by the journal such as a black and white photograph of yourself, a brief biographical sketch, an abstract, and a curriculum vitae. Include your name, address, telephone number, job title, and affiliation. Write a brief, to-the-point letter to accompany the manuscript.

Mail the manuscript in a padded mailer or sturdy manilla envelope. It is best to send it certified with a return receipt requested.

After you have mailed the manuscript, the waiting begins. Turnaround time for review varies widely. Check the information given by the journal you have submitted the manuscript to for an idea of when to expect a response. Most editors will acknowledge receipt, or your return receipt card will verify that the manuscript reached its destination. The review process is described in an excellent article by Swanson and McCloskey (45).

Major reasons for rejection include: subject already covered in a scheduled issue; subject too technical, inaccurate or undocumented; poor research design; faulty methodology; nursing aspects not well described; content unimportant; you have tried to convert a speech into an article; the conclusion is unwarranted by the data; the material has been published elsewhere; or the material is poorly presented (45). Some editors will write you a letter giving you a critique of the manuscript, whereas from others you will receive only a form letter or a polite thank you and please try again. Occasionally, rejection letters can be somewhat demoralizing if not downright caustic, so develop a thick skin, learn from any helpful comments you can glean, reread and rewrite if necessary, and try again. Hints on handling rejection are included in a very useful article by two seasoned writers (46).

Summary

Research should not be neglected by nurses in advanced practice roles. As mavericks and risk takers in nursing, they can be leaders in clinical research as well. The field of nursing is so fertile that a rich harvest can be gleaned from the bounty of everyday practice in terms of researchable topics and issues that affect and shape the course of health care now and will affect and shape it in the future. Research will provide a sound rationale for what nurses in advanced practice roles do and what they say they do.

REFERENCES

1. Gortner, S.R., Fisher, S.G., Rugg, J., Hubbard, S. & McGuire, D. (1979). The three faces of teaching research issues. In: Power: Nursing's Challenge for Change Papers presented at the 51st Convention, Honolulu, Hawaii, June 9-14, 1978. Kansas City, MO: American Nurses' Association, p. 117.
2. Shipley, S.B. (1980). The practitioner's role in nursing research. Association of Operating Room Nurses (AORN) Journal 31:102-103.
3. Carnegie, M.E. (1976). Historical Perspectives of Nursing Re-

search. Boston, MA: Boston University Mugar Memorial Library Nursing Archives. pp. 1-14.
4. Brown, E.L. (1949). Nursing for the Future. New York: Russell Sage. p. 100.
5. Smoyak, S.A. (1976). Is practice responding to research? American Journal of Nursing 76:1146-1150.
6. Joint Committee on Nursing Research and Studies. (1952). Research in nursing - philosophy and plan of action. American Journal of Nursing 52:601-603.
7. Simmons, L.W. & Henderson, V. (1964). Nursing Research: Survey and Assessment. New York: Appleton-Century-Crofts.
8. Fox, D.J. (1966). Fundamentals of Research in Nursing. New York: Appleton-Century-Crofts.
9. Abdellah, F.G. & Levine, E. (1965). Better Patient Care through Nursing Research. New York: Macmillan.
10. Carnegie, M.E., op. cit., p. 23.
11. Nursing Data Review (1992). New York: National League for Nursing
12. Jacox, A.K. & Norris, C.M. (Eds.) (1977). Organizing for Independent Nursing Practice. New York: Appleton-Century-Crofts. pp. 205-206.
13. O'Toole, A.W. (1979). The expanded role: Issues and opportunities for nursing. In: Power Nursing's Challenge for Change. Papers Presented at the 51st Convention, Honolulu, Hawaii, June 9-14. Kansas City, MO: American Nurses' Association. p. 60.
14. Barnard, K.E. (1980). Knowledge for practice: Directions for the future. Nursing Research 29:208-212.
15. Wilson, H.S. (1992). Identifying problems for clinical research to create a nursing tapestry. Image 91(3):64-65.
16. Johnson, B.K. (1991). How to ask research questions in clinical practice. American Journal of Nursing 91(3):64-65.
17. Ford, L.C. (1979). A nurse for all settings: The nurse practitioner. Nursing Outlook 27:520-521.
18. Jacox, A.K. & Norris, C.M. (Eds.). op. cit., pp. 209-210.
19. Ibid., p. 212.
20. Cronenwett, L.R. (1986). The research role of the clinical nurse

specialist. Journal of Nursing Administration 16(4):10-11.
21. Brodish, M.S., Chamings, P.A. & Tranbarger, R.E. (1987). Fostering a research focus for the clinical nurse specialist. Clinical Nurse Specialist 1(3):99-l04.
22. Gortner, S.R., Fisher, S.G., Rugg, J., Hubbard, S. & McGuire, D., op. cit., pp. 118-123.
23. Martin, J.P. (1990). Implementing the research role of the clinical nurse specialist — one institution's approach. Clinical Nurse Specialist 4(3):137-140.24.
24. Stanford, D. (1989). Nurse practitioner research: Issues in practice and theory. The Nurse Practitioner 12(1):64-65, 68, 72, 74-75.
24a Douglas, S., Hill, M.N. & Cameron, E.M. (1989). Clinical nurse specialist: A facilitator for clinical research. Clinical Nurse Specialist 3(1):12-15.
25. Denyes, M.J., O'Connor, N.A., Oakley, D. & Ferguson, S. (1989). Integrating nursing theory, practice, and research through collaborative research. Journal of Advanced Nursing 14:141-145.
26. Notter, L.E. (1975). The case for nursing research. Nursing Outlook 23:760-763.
27. Taylor, R., Crabtree, M.K., Renwanz-Boye, A., Perry, B. & Thrallkill, A. (1990). A collaborative approach to nursing research: Part I: The process. Journal of the American Academy of Nurse Practitioners 2(4):140-145.
28. Crabtree, M.K., Renwanz-Boyle, A., Perry, B., Taylor, R. & Thrallkill, A. (1990). A collaborative approach to nursing research: Part II: The findings. Journal of the American Academy of Nurse Practitioners 2(4):146-152.
28a Johnson, J.E. (1979). Translating research to practice. In: Power: Nursing's Challenge for Change. Papers Presented at the 5lst convention, Honolulu, Hawaii, June 9-14, 1978. Kansas City, MO: American Nurses' Association, p. 125.
28b Barnard, K.E., op. cit.
29. Miller, J.R. & Messenger, S.R. (1978). Obstacles to applying nursing research findings. American Journal of Nursing 78:632-634.
30. King, D., Barnard, K.E. & Hoehn, R. (1981). Disseminating the results of nursing research. Nursing Research 29:164-169.

31. Hickey, M. (1990). The role of the clinical nurse specialist in the research utilization process. Clinical Nurse Specialist 4(2):93-96.
32. Stetler, C.B. & Mimaggio, G. (1991). Research utilization among clinical nurse specialists. Clinical Nurse Specialist 5(3):151-155.
33. Johnson, J.E., op. cit., pp. 125-126.
34. Ibid., p. 133.
35. Stetler, C.B. & Marram, G. (1976). Evaluating research findings for applicability in practice. Nursing Outlook 24:559-563.
36. Styles, M.M. (1978). Why publish? Image 10:28-32.
37. Diers, D. (1980). Why write? Why publish? Image 13:3-8.
38. Swanson, E.A., McCloskey, J.C. & Bodensteiner A. (1991). Publishing opportunities for nurses: A comparison of 92 U.S. journals. Image 23(1):33-38.
39. Grace, H.K. (1980). For the refereed journal. Nursing Outlook 28:423.
40. Lewis, E.P. (1980). A peerless publication. Editorial. Nursing Outlook 28:225-226.
41. Swanson et al. (1991). op cit.
42. Lewis, E.P. (1982). For the nurse writer's bookshelf. American Journal of Nursing 82(7):1116-1118.
43. Hodgman, E.C. (1980). On writing and writing workshops. Nursing Outlook 28:366-371.
44. Johnson, S.H. (1989). Finding time to write within a busy CNS schedule. Momentum 7(2):1; 3-4.
45. Swanson, E. & McCloskey, J.C. (1982). The manuscript review process of nursing journals. Image 14:72-76.
46. Gay, J.T. & Edgil, A.E. (1989). When your manuscript is rejected. Nursing and Health Care 10(8):459-461.

BIBLIOGRAPHY

Blancett, S.S. (1991). Who is entitled to authorship? Nurse Educator 16(5):3.

Blancett, S.S. (1991). The ethics of writing and publishing. Journal of

Nursing Administration 21(5):31-36.
Blancett, S.S. (1988). The process and politics of writing for publication. Clinical Nurse Specialist 2(3):113-117.
Blosnan, J., Kovalesky, A. & Lewis, E.P. (1980). Perishing while publishing. Nursing Outlook 28:688-690.
Brooten, D.E. (1986). Who's on first? Nursing Research 35:259.
Boykoff, S.L. (1989). Coauthorship: Collaboration without conflict. American Journal of Nursing 89(9):1164.
Camillieri, R. (1987). Six ways to write right. Image 19:210-212.
Dixon, J. (1982). Developing the evaluation component of a grant application. Nursing Outlook 30:122-127.
Edgil, A.E. & Gay, J.T. (1983). Nurses can write for publication. Journal of Obstetric, Gynecologic and Neonatal Nursing 12:231-235.
Fitzpatrick, J.J. (1990). The power of the written word. Applied Nursing Research 3(1)1.
Fitzpatrick, J.J. (1988). The joys and triumphs of clinical nursing research. Applied Nursing Research 1(3):107-108.
Hanson, S.M.H. (1988). Collaborative research and authorship credit: Beginning guidelines. Nursing Research 37:49-52.
Hanson, S.M.H. (1988). Write on. American Journal of Nursing 88:482-483.
Hodgson, C. (1989). Tips on writing successful grant proposals. The Nurse Practitioner 14(2):44; 46; 49; 52; 54.
Holmstrom, L.L. & Burgess, A.W. (1982). Low-cost research: A project on a shoestring. Nursing Research 31:123-125.
Jimenez, S.L.M. (1991). Consumer journalism: A unique nursing opportunity. Image: 23(1):47-49.
Johnson, S.H. (1982). Selecting a journal for your manuscript. Nursing and Health Care 3(5):258-263.
Kelly, J.A. & Gay, J.T. (1990). Grantsmanship: The process/the art. Nursing and Health Care 11(7):346-352.
Kemp, C. (1991). A practical approach to writing successful grant proposals. The Nurse Practitioner 16(11):51; 55-56.
Kilby, S.A., Rupp, L.F., Fishel, C.C. & Brecht, M. (1991). Changes in nursing's periodical literature: 1975-1985. Nursing Outlook 39(2):82-86.

Parse, R.R. (1990). Making more out of less...Publishing the same manuscript in more than one journal. Nursing Science Quarterly 2(4):155.

Perry, S.E. (1989). Misuse of common words. Research in Nursing and Health 12(3):iii-iv.

Publication Manual of the American Psychological Association. 3rd. ed. (1983). Washington, DC: American Psychological Association.

Robinson, A.M. & Notter, L.E. (1982). Clinical Writing for Health Professionals. Bowie, MD: Brady.

Sexton, D.L. (1982). Developing skills in grant writing. Nursing Outlook 30:31-38.

Strickland, O.L., Burgess, A.W., Oberst, M.T. & Kim, H.S. (1987). Private sector support of nursing research. Nursing Research 36:253-256.

Tornquist, E.M., Funk, S.G. & Champagne, M.T. (1989). Writing research reports for clinical audiences. Western Journal of Nursing Research 11(5):576-582.

Trussell, P., Brandt, A. & Knapp, S. (1981). Using Nursing Research: Discovery, Analysis, and Interpretation. Wakefield, MA: Nursing Resources.

Turabian, L.L. (1973). A Manual for Writers, 4th ed. Chicago: University of Chicago Press.

Waltz, C.F., Nelson, B. & Chambers, S.B. (1985). Assigning publication credits. Nursing Outlook 33:233-238.

White, J. (1986). Nurses who publish journal articles. Nursing Outlook 34:225-226.

White, V. (1983). Grant Proposals that Succeeded. New York: Plenum.

9
Negotiating an Employment Contract

Introduction

One of the most crucial tasks of the nurse is preparing for and negotiating the employment contract. All too often students are so proud — and rightly so — of their accomplishments upon completing a master's program that the process of contract negotiation does not get all the attention it should.

Negotiating a "position package" is the synthesis of the entire educational experience. Here the philosophies of nursing and of specialty care must mesh with the reality of the work world. Nursing theory and nursing science must find fruition in a fertile work environment. Assertive techniques and leadership strategies must be put to the crucial test. If the nurse does not "sell" herself/himself during the negotiating process and behaves in a nonassertive, passive manner, future dealings may be impaired.

Developing a Portfolio

The first step in preparing for negotiating a contract is to prepare a portfolio. This should include one's written philosophies of nursing and specialty care (not for the eyes of the employer but to help the nurse clarify her/his own views so that the negotiations can be dealt with from strength), a resume or CV, a written description of the type of position wanted, documents such as licenses, and a thoroughly researched paper about the salary desired. The purpose of a portfolio is to assemble *all* relevant information about one's self in one place. This becomes the source from which current resumes are developed (1).

Developing and Writing Philosophies of Nursing and Specialty Care

One of the first steps toward securing the right position with the most favorable conditions is to have thought out and written clearly articulated, succinct philosophies of nursing and specialty care. All practitioners and clinical specialists would surely state that they are seeking a position in a place where the philosophical position is compatible with their own, since philosophical differences have often been a source of disenchantment with a position. When that occurs, is it because the nurse has not solidified a philosophy and therefore cannot deal adequately with specific points in the discussion during the employment interview? To clarify such points, the practitioner or clinician should *write out* philosophies of nursing and specialty care.

The philosophy of nursing has to do with issues of independence, autonomy, and professional growth potential within the work setting. It should be limited to a maximum of three pages. It should address the topics of person, environment, health, and nursing as discussed in Chapter 1.

The written philosophy is not meant as a lofty exercise but rather as a translation of basic concepts into the "real world" setting. Reflection on the concept of person leads to a variety of questions about the prospective position. Is active participation by the client and mutual goal setting encouraged? Is equal emphasis placed on psychosocial needs as on physical ones? What are the supports and/or constraints to desired scope of practice in the environment? Does the setting allow the nurse sufficient time for health teaching? How much control does the nurse have in the scheduling of clients? Is there opportunity to work with families and with other health care professionals? What are the opportunities for advancement?

One's philosophy of health also translates into practical concerns. Is the focus of the employing agency geared toward cure, health maintenance, health promotion, or a balance among these three levels of health care?

A *philosophy of specialty care,* emanating from the general nursing philosophy, should be written next and evaluated for consistency and logic. The philosophy of specialty care is best limited to one page. It should focus on the specifics of the specialty care component of health care delivery such as scope of practice, referral network, relationships with other health care professionals, and clinical research.

The Resume

The resume is an extremely important document since it is most often the first thing a prospective employer evaluates. A resume is a summary of all the pertinent facts about one's background and professional experiences (1).

It is important to differentiate between a professional resume and a curriculum vitae. The primary purpose of a resume is to entice an employer to grant an interview for a position. As such, it needs to be adapted for a variety of potential readers. The style and format vary for different situations (2). Sometimes a different resume must be developed for each position sought.

The basic information regarding personal data, educational endeavors, professional experience, and professional activities must be included, but the resume can be stylized to emphasize the "fit" between your background and the person the employer is seeking or may be encouraged to seek even if she/he was not actively advertising a specific position. The resume can spell out various responsibilities and highlight functions of previous jobs, and can delineate what the job seeker has to offer. In short, the purpose of a resume is to attract the employer's attention and to make him/her anxious to hire you. Your resume is your entree into the work world. You may be a fantastic conversationalist, but you may not get the chance for an interview if your resume does not "sell" you.

The Curriculum Vitae

The curriculum vitae, on the other hand, "is a more rigidly prescribed document designated for use in the highly structural world of academe" (2). Since the CV is used almost exclusively for presenting one's qualifications for an academic position, including that of consultant or researcher, it is not modified as is the resume. The CV follows a standard format and should include personal data, education, experience, research, grants, honors and awards, professional memberships, and publications, research presentation, and invited papers (3). The CV is a chronicle of scholarly achievements. Articles published in nonprofessional magazines or talks given to community groups, for example, may not be appropriate for the CV but may be very relevant to the resume if a facet of the position sought involves public relations (2).

The CV should be prepared and presented if the practitioner or clinical specialist is seeking an academic position. If she or he desires to obtain a clinical position, the resume is the appropriate document to prepare for one's portfolio. If the position sought is a joint clinical and academic appointment, the nurse must be prepared to be interviewed by service persons and academics.

It is not only the content of the CV or resume which is important, but also its style and manner of presentation. Besides knowing the difference between a resume and CV, the practitioner or clinical specialist should know what to include or exclude within the general categories mentioned earlier. It is to your disadvantage to exclude important information about your experiences and achievements. It is just as serious to "pad" your CV or resume with insignificant or nonprofessional activities.

It is suggested that the practitioner/clinician prepare a draft copy of the CV or resume and submit it to a professional agency or to an experienced academician/clinician for feedback before preparing the final document. Considering the importance of this document to one's professional career, professional advice is time and money well spent.

Next, the appearance of the CV or resume must be considered. The most highly qualified scholar/clinician will tarnish her/his image if the CV or resume is unattractive. The CV or resume should be professionally typed and reproduced on sturdy 8½ x 11 bond paper. This document should contain no typing errors, erasure marks, misspellings, syntax errors, or uneven margins, and should be cleanly typed. A word to the wise: proofread your CV or resume before copies are reproduced or, better yet, have someone else do it. Any errors will reflect upon you, not on your typist. A word processor/computer is immensely helpful in producing a CV/resume.

Often advanced practitioners are reluctant to spend the money to have a CV or resume professionally typed. This is an instance of being penny wise and pound foolish. Twenty-five to fifty dollars spent on this document could be the key to the right job with more money, and could well yield thousands of dollars more in the long run. The same advice holds true for dressing appropriately for the job interview. Appearance, whether it be yours or that of your resume or CV, does make a definite impression upon a potential employer and/or interviewer.

The Position Description

Clinical specialists and nurse practitioners (nurses who are advanced practitioners) often find themselves seeking positions for which there are no established guidelines or parameters. A general position description written by the nurse practitioner or clinical specialist is another document to be included in one's professional portfolio. This document should be shared with potential employers. The position description specifies your views about your areas of responsibility, qualifications, and functions (4). If you are seeking a position not specifically advertised in a journal or newspaper, for example, then a written statement of what you hope to do and have to offer is a good idea. Advertised positions usually have a job description which has been written by the employing agency. The advanced practitioner should definitely ask to see this document, if one is available.

"The job description is essential because it states the function for which the nursing staff member is held accountable, the performance expectations, and how that contribution is to be measured" (5). A job description has several uses. First, it serves as a starting point from which to negotiate the specifics of a given position. Second, it clarifies areas of potential misunderstanding between employer and employee related to anticipated roles and responsibilities (6). The practitioner or clinician must ascertain that the roles and responsibilities fall within the scope of practice prescribed by the professional organizations and the state's nurse practice act.

Documents

It is also useful to collect all pertinent documents regarding your professional career and include them in the portfolio for your personal use. Include copies of professional licenses, evidence of certification, transcripts, malpractice insurance policies, and your state's nurse practice act (1).

Salary

Last but not least, you need to do some extensive preparation regarding salary requirements *before* going for a position interview. Jacox and Norris present a useful rule of thumb for the determination of salary range (7). It is first necessary to determine the gross income generated by your services. For example, if you see one client an hour at a charge of $40 per visit, you will generate $1,400 at 35 hours per week or $72,800 per year. Subtract 40 percent for overhead, medical back-up, and consultation costs, and the resulting figure should be within a reasonable salary range.

When the nurse does this kind of salary determination it should be easy to overcome the temptation to timidly accept any salary offered by the employer. Facts and figures put you in the driver's seat in the negotiation process. You should also be aware of the salary range in the area where employment is being sought. Salaries may vary greatly with geographic area.

The salary figure quoted should be considered in light of the total benefits package and how important it is to you. Fringe benefits such as health insurance, retirement or pension plan, sick leave, and holiday time can add approximately 50% percent to the base salary (6). A higher salary without fringe benefits may be worth less than a lower one with fringe benefits. Other fringe benefits to consider are tuition reimbursement, certification and licensure costs, time off with pay for professional development, malpractice insurance, mileage reimbursement, secretarial services including help with publications and research, and reimbursement for necessary equipment.

Don't forget to consider the process for determining periodic salary increments and the amounts involved. Is a cost of living increase automatically provided? Is there a union to which nurse practitioners or clinical nurse specialists can belong? If so, what are the dues and the specifics of the union contract? Is it a labor union or professional union contract? How is meritorious service rewarded by the employer? What are the methods and processes used for evaluation? Who evaluates you? Has a system of peer review been established? Wolf (6) suggests keeping a record, with cost-benefit analyses, of clients seen and clinical activities such as research projects, for use in the process of on-going salary renegotiation.

Almost every salary is negotiable — even if you aren't negotiating the employer is. "Low aspirations can actually disqualify you from jobs ... If you put a small price on yourself, that's about what the employer will think you are worth" (8). Take the initiative and name a high salary. You can always lower your aspirations, but once you have named your rock-bottom salary it is impossible to command a higher price.

Salary negotiations should take place at the end of the interviewing stage. There is a sound rationale behind this timing. "Until the employer has made up his or her mind to hire you, you aren't worth anything to that person. By delaying money talk, you can develop your strengths, communicate your accomplishments, and show how you can meet the other person's needs so that when the time comes to discuss money, you are actually worth more in his/her eyes" (8).

The Position Interview

Much has been written about the position interview and little about the very important steps that prepare one for it. If you have done the preparation, the interview should go smoothly. Your philosophy will direct and guide the general questions you want to ask of the employer, and you will be prepared to answer any questions asked of you by the employer. The employer's view of person, environment, health, and nursing as well as of specialty care must be ascertained and compared to yours to evaluate compatibility. This task is definitely easier when the questions asked of the employer are generated specifically from the philosophy of the prospective employee. Areas of essential agreement must be identified first. If there is incompatibility in areas you have identified as crucial to your basic philosophy (such as time for teaching and for illness prevention), negotiations should center around those issues. If agreement is not possible, that may be sufficient reason to terminate the negotiations no matter how attractive other aspects of the position may be.

Assuming that you have had several interviews and that more than one position is basically in tune with your philosophy, you can prioritize the answers of potential employers to the questions you asked them about philosophy by dividing the answers into positive or negative aspects and using them as additional data for comparing one position with another. These comparisons are best made after all the interviews when you have time to reflect. Since positions are rarely offered outright at the time of an interview, there should be sufficient time to weigh all the factors carefully.

The resume or CV will serve as a concise outline from which you can elaborate about your education and experience. The job description can serve as the specific point of departure for negotiation of specific roles and responsibilities. Your preparation regarding salary and fringe benefits should give you a comfortable range within which to bargain. Be prepared also to meet with a variety of persons during the interview process. These may include the agency administrator, the nurse director, or physicians, and may occur at different times.

After you've done your homework, proceed with the interviews in a positive manner. Be assertive and put your best foot forward. Dress appropriately, neatly, and professionally. Look at the interviews as learning experiences. Even if you don't accept the position or are not offered it, what you learn from it will help you in future interviews.

Final terms of negotiation should be incorporated into a written document which is open to annual renegotiation. Through the process of prepared negotiation, the practitioner or clinical specialist will be in the best possible position for career satisfaction, which will benefit both employee and employer.

Autonomy and Accountability

Mauksch identified four critical issues related to the role and practice of advanced practitioners: autonomy, accountability, client advocacy, and self-actualization (9). Autonomy and accountability are particularly relevant when considering a professional position. The potential employee should carefully consider his/her position regarding these issues and explore them with potential employers during the interview.

Autonomy and accountability are interrelated and logically flow from one's philosophy. A job must have the potential for both if you are going to be able to practice as you were educated. Autonomy means that you will have a feeling of independence and self-direction which will enable you to be accountable both to yourself and your clients without an intermediary. Autonomy does not mean that the practitioner works in isolation without the benefit of medical and/or other health professional consultation and collaboration, but rather that she or he has the freedom to practice at the maximum potential permitted legally within the scope of nursing practice. Accountability means the assumption of responsibility inherent in the exercise of one's profession.

Summary

Preparing for employment negotiations includes developing written philosophies of nursing and specialty care. A CV or resume should be compiled and professionally typed. The professional portfolio should also include a position description and related professional documents. An acceptable salary range and fringe benefits should be determined before the interview. The documents prepared for the portfolio serve as guidelines and focus of the interview process. This initial negotiation sets the tone for all future relationships with the prospective employer.

REFERENCES

1. Edmunds, R. (1980). Developing a marketing portfolio. The Nurse Practitioner 5:41-46.
2. Newcomb, J. & Murphy, P.A. (1979). The curriculum vitae - what it is and what it is not. Nursing Outlook 27:580-583.
3. Van Leunen, M.C. (1978). A Handbook for Scholars. New York: Alfred A. Knopf.
4. Edmunds, M. (1979). The position description. The Nurse Practitioner 4:45-47.
5. Brockenshire, A. & Hattstaedt, M.J.O. (1980). Revising job descriptions: A consensus approach. Supervisor Nurse 11:16-20.
6. Wolf, G.A. (1980). Negotiating an employment contract. The Nurse Practitioner 5:55, 60.
7. Jacox, A.K. & Norris, C.M. (1977). Organizing for Independent Nursing Practice. New York: Appleton-Century-Crofts.
8. Chastain, D. (1981). How to play your hand for a salary. New York Times, Oct. 11, Section 12:60.
9. Mauksch, I.G. (1978). Critical issues of the nurse practitioner movement. The Nurse Practitioner 3:35-36.

BIBLIOGRAPHY

Aimes, A.., Adkins, S., et al. (1992). Assessing work retention issues. Journal of Nursing Administration 22:37-41.

Collins, M. (1991). First impressions made in interviews. The American Nurse 23(3):24.

Collins, M. (1991). Resume is key to getting a job. The American Nurse 23(2):18.

Dadich, K.A. (1992). Your resume. Health Care Trends and Transitions 3(2):20-24.

Fisher, A.B. (1988). If we're so smart, why aren't we rich? Savvy, August:36-38, 84-86.

Houlihan, R. (1991). Interviewing tips for the 90's nurse. Massachusetts Nurse 61(8):4.

Jones, A.G. (1991). Gaining control of the CNS role through written contracts. Clinical Nurse Specialist 5(2):101-104.
Kalisch, P.A. & Kalisch, B.J. (1987). The Changing Image of the Nurse. Menlo Park, CA: Wesley Publishing Company.
McCloskey, J.C. (1990). Two requirements for job contentment: Autonomy and social integration. Image 22:140-143.
Sape, G.P. (1985). Coping with comparable worth. Harvard Business Review 63(3):145-152.
Sands, J.K. (1991). Avoiding the pitfalls of job hunting. Healthcare Trends & Transitions 3(1):52-55.
Shamansky, S. (1981). Marketing nurse practitioner services. The Nurse Practitioner 6:42, 50-51.
Styles, M.M. (1985). The uphill battle for comparable worth. Nursing Outlook 33(3):128-137.
Sullivan, J.A., Dachelet, C.Z., Sultz, H.A., Henry, O.M. & Carrol, H.D. (1978). Overcoming barriers to the employment and utilization of the nurse practitioner. American Journal of Public Health 68:1097-1103.
Tyler, L. (1990). Watch out for "red flags" on a job interview. Hospitals 64(14).
Vogel, D. & Jackson, P. (1992). The interview. Reflections from the recruiter's side of the desk. Healthcare Trends & Transitions 3(4): 24-26.
Walters, J.A. (1987). An innovative method of job interviewing. The Journal of Nursing Administration 17(5):25-29.
Winstead-Fry, P. (1990). Career Planning: A Nurse's Guide to Career Advancement. New York: National League for Nursing.

10

Economics of the Roles

Introduction

When Lucille Kinlein hung out her shingle announcing her independent nursing practice, she was unorthodox in more than one respect. Nurses have long been relegated to economically dependent roles within the context of a free enterprise health care delivery system. Caught up in such a tradition, nurses have been slow to enter the economic world of the twentieth century. Kinlein was a risk-taker in an economic sense, and those who followed her example were willing to brave the economic uncertainties of the new role. In this chapter, we will explore the various modes of being a nurse in advanced practice from a business perspective.

Independent Practice

One of the hazards inherent in independent practice is economic uncertainty. The public is unaccustomed to paying nurses directly for their services. Furthermore, third-party reimbursement mechanisms for nurses are still not well developed, so nurses must rely on associations with physicians or on special circumstances such as rural health clinic status in order to be directly reimbursed, or special populations such as nursing home residents or recipients of Medicaid.

In 1973, when the first American Nurses Association Committee was established to consider independent nursing practice, the issue of third-part reimbursement received top priority. Economic issues are still among those most important to nurses launching independent or group nursing practices.

Planning for Independent Practice

Launching an independent practice requires far more than developing a philosophy of care, a plan to implement that philosophy in practice, and means for evaluation (1). Independent practice requires thoughtful planning for its business aspects.

Assessment

Simplistic as it may sound, setting up a private practice should follow the steps of the nursing process. First, you will need to spend a considerable amount of time assessing the needs of your proposed target client population, formulating and/or articulating the philosophy, objectives, and scope of your practice, preparing protocols, collecting information on how you will fit in and work with other health care providers, and surveying possible locations.

Some of the components of the assessment process are addressed in other chapters: philosophy and scope of practice; community needs; and interdisciplinary relationships. Here we will concentrate on the business and economic aspects. Exploring the business aspects might include gathering information on the costs of renting space, telephone service, advertising, any necessary equipment to rent or purchase, disposable or reusable supplies, record-keeping materials, and various means for financing a small business.

Acquiring business skills is very helpful for the nurse who is setting up a private practice. Short courses, workshops, and college classes on business are available (2). Little has yet been done to incorporate courses in business and economics into undergraduate or graduate nursing programs (3), although future programs may well include them. In order to maximize the potential of nurses prepared to practice as independent providers, perhaps these nurses need "some basic training in being an entrepreneur"(3).

Selecting a Site. The location for your practice may be critical to its success. Unless you plan a practice which encompasses only home visits, you will need space in which to interview and perhaps examine your clients. You may be fortunate enough to have suitable space in your own residence. Some advanced practitioners have been able to convert one room into an adequate office and consulting room, either in their apartment or private residence. It is important to check zoning laws, however, so as not to violate any regulations. If it is not feasible to use your home, or if your home is not central to your target population, you will have to look for space elsewhere since access for your clients is of utmost importance.

When looking for space, consider proximity to public transportation, available parking space, and choose a building that has an elevator and is accessible to those with disabilities (4, 5). Consider whether or not the neighborhood is a safe one for you and your clients, and whether or not it is one that will attract clients for you. If your target population is older people, consider locating near a senior citizen's housing project. If it is a low-income ethnic population, select a site in such a neighborhood. It may be possible for you to share an office suite with other providers. Perhaps a local dentist owns or rents a building with two or more offices and would be willing to rent one to you. You may also consider group practice with other nurses or with physicians or other health care providers.

The amount of space you anticipate needing is an important consideration. Will you require a waiting area? Will you need an office and an examining room? A bathroom is probably a necessity, even if it is shared with other tenants.

Rent and the terms of the lease are the next considerations. Assess the rent in light of an security deposit required and your ability to carry the costs until your practice is sufficiently established to cover expenses. It is wise to have an attorney review the lease for you (5).

Once you have secured a place, you will need to equip and furnish it. Unless you are fortunate enough to be renting a furnished suite, joining an established group practice, or can make arrangements to buy out a previous tenant or another practice, you need to assess realistically the costs of making your office functional.

Office and waiting room furniture and accessories such as lamps, rugs, and curtains are often available in secondhand stores or even from your own household, family, and friends. A computer is one item you may need to buy new. If you require examining room equipment, costs can escalate quickly. Comparison shop, check sources for used equipment, and do a thorough search before you decide on new equipment. A new examining table can cost hundreds of dollars, examination stools and lamps can cost up to a hundred or more dollars each, and miscellaneous equipment such as a side cabinet, otoscope, ophthalmoscope, eye chart, tuning forks, sphygmomanometer, and stethoscope are all very expensive. Be sure to include costs of disposable items such as tongue blades, paper for the examining table, drapes for clients (some nurses in advanced practice have made their own washable table covers and drapes), and office and record-keeping supplies. If you will be using equipment that can be resterilized, how will you accomplish this? Will you need laundry services of any sort? If you require laboratory services, these must be arranged, and it is possible that, as an independent nurse, you may encounter difficulties in doing so (6). Can you meet new Centers for Disease Control (CDC) and Occupational Safety and Health Administration (OSHA) regulations?

Business Arrangements. When selecting a name for your practice, consider one that will convey who and what you are, one that people will remember, one that is not offensive in any way or that will put people off, and one that does not duplicate the names of other groups or individuals. You may want to incorporate. In that event, your attorney will assist you in researching names of corporations already in use in the state. Incorporating will protect your home and family from any malpractice suit (7). After you have selected a name for your practice, visit several printing services for estimates and have business cards, stationery, and perhaps brochures prepared.

In planning for telephone services, inquire about advertising in the yellow pages, answering services, business rates, and any deposit or installation fees required. Nurses in private practice have even had to fight for the right to have a business phone listing in the telephone directory's white pages (8).

Once you have a location and have made it functional, you will need to advertise for clients. Advertising requires a lot of public relations work. You may choose to advertise in the local paper. A mailing of brochures to prospective groups or organizations can be helpful. You will need to make yourself kown to other providers: health care professionals, clergy, social service agencies, senior citizen's centers, childbirth education groups, or whatever is appropriate to your particular practice.

Financial Planning. Careful financial planning is critical in setting up your own business. Your assessment will provide you with the data on start-up costs. Beginning an independent practice can cost from a few hundred to several thousand dollars, but it can be done on shoestring with careful planning (10). Allowing for inflation, it is probable that you can plan on at least several hundred dollars as an absolute minimum (see Table 10.1). In addition to the actual costs involved in equipping and supplying an office, getting office supplies and a telephone, advertising, and so on, it is imperative to plan for expenses that will be ongoing, such as rent, until you can expect the practice to be self-supporting (9) (see Table 10.2). If you plan to devote full time to the practice, you also need to plan for your living costs until the practice generates an income for you over and above business costs (2) (see Table 10.3).

When you have determined the initial costs and business and personal expenses for the first few months of practice, it is time to evaluate your assets and debits to determine if you can afford to go into private practice. If your anticipated start-up costs exceed your resources, other sources of funds must be sought. Consider small business loans. The assistance of a banker or financial officer versed in the economic aspects of starting a small business can be invaluable. Other sources of funds include: personal loans, private investment companies, government lending programs, small business investment companies,

Table 10.1 Start-up Costs for Independent Practice*

Rent for first and last months
Deposit on rental
Stationery supplies and office forms
Telephone installation and deposit (one or more lines)
Telephone answering machine or answering service
Incorporation fees
Equipment for office and examining room — probably include computer, copy machine, fax machine
Laboratory equipment including microscope, Glucometer®
Supplies for examinations and record keeping
Advertising: brochures, ads, mailings, newsletter, business cards, signs, yellow pages
Utility deposits and/or meter installation fees
Fees such as licensure
Any decorating or remodeling costs
Malpractice insurance
Attorney, accountant, architect fees
Incidentals: petty cash, coffee, tea bags, cups, toilet paper, paper towels, etc.
Checking account — cost of having checks printed, any service charges
Educational materials for clients
Typewriter or computer supplies
Financing costs
Contingency fund (minimum of 5% of budget)

* Adapted from Dalton (4), Pearson (9), and Nichols and Nichols (10)

business development companies, loan companies, and equipment finance companies (11). Since interest charges, fees, loan terms, and collateral statements can be very complex, it is prudent to seek professional advice.

Once you have financing for your business, the next step is to plan short- and long-term budgets. Predictions as to financial viability must be based on the experiences of others, so search the literature and talk with health care providers in your area. Be realistic and conservative in

Table 10.2 Operating Expenses

Rent or mortgage
Utilities: light, heat, water
Telephone
Telephone answering service, if needed
Maintenance: cleaning services and cleaning supplies and equipment; maintenance cost for office equipment
Disposables: office supplies, examination room and laboratory supplies, miscellaneous such as coffee, tea, etc.
Laboratory fees
Advertising: ads, brochures, newsletter, yellow pages
Laundry services — lab coats, scrub suits, towels, gowns, table covers
Malpractice insurance and other insurance fees; business taxes, Social Security
Accountant fees
Postage
Checks: service for checking account
Duplication of records for referral

---

your projections for break-even and profit points.

Budget planning necessitates fee setting. Fees reflect how you value your services. At the same time, they must be realistic in relation to the means of your target population and in line with the fees charged by other providers. Some nurses choose to have sliding scale fees (7). Your method of fee collection will also affect income. If the fees are paid at the time of service, you will eliminate the time lag between the visit and payment, and your bookkeeping will be easier. Deferred billing may sometimes be a reasonable approach to assure that service is not denied to those who need it. Persons on fixed incomes may find a flexible payment scheme helpful. It is realistic to plan on some uncollectible fees.

The next step, unless you have some expertise in bookkeeping and accounting, is to seek the services of an accountant. You will need to set up a bookkeeping system to account for all income and output. You may need federal and state identification numbers for reporting

Table 10.3 Personal Expenses*

Rent, condominium fees and/or mortgage and taxes
Food
Insurance: health, life, property
Car insurance and taxes, licenses, operating expenses
Upkeep of home
Clothing
Utilities: gas, water, electricity; oil, wood or coal (for heat)
Telephone
Any outstanding loan or credit payments
Taxes: federal, state, local
Medical, dental expenses
Dues, subscriptions to journals, licensure and registration fees, travel to professional meetings, maintenance of licensure and certification, continuing education courses
Recreation: movies, travel, plays, concerts, vacations, eating out
Miscellaneous: newspapers, cosmetics, OTC drugs, laundry, cleaning supplies, personal hygiene products, postage, gifts, educational expense
Pets: care and feeding

* Adapted from Edmunds (2)

purposes. Some cities and also some states require a business license. You probably will have some mechanism for billing third parties for allowable cases and to assist clients in obtaining private insurance reimbursement. Medicare and Medicaid reimbursement mechanisms require considerable paperwork.

If you decide to employ a receptionist or an assistant of some sort, you will need to develop payroll protocols and comply with regulations for tax withholding and social security payments. It is best to have completely separate bank accounts and bookkeeping for your business and personal accounts (12). Once you are actually using the bookkeeping and client record systems you planned so carefully, you may find they are too cumbersome or time consuming or incomplete. With the best planning in the world, systems cannot be perfected until they are actually used.

Evaluation

Once your office is ready, your advertising under way, and your bookkeeping systems in place, you are ready to begin. As Lucille Kinlein put it, "I sat back and waited for my first client to come" (13). After all the planning and anticipation, the big day has arrived — you are an independent practitioner.

Evaluation and quality improvement are important and often neglected aspects of independent practice. These were discussed in detail in Chapter Seven. Evaluating your practice should be ongoing. It is possible to structure your practice so as to elicit input from other nurse peers on a periodic basis. If you are in a group nursing practice, you can get input from one another by holding clinical conferences and perhaps meetings on office management as well (4). Setting regular times for evaluation and review will assure that these meetings occur. Soliciting feedback from clients will help you assess which services they most value, how best to reach the potential client population, and how to be most responsive to your clients' perceptions of their needs. Furthermore, evaluation, quality improvement, and outcome measures will provide data to support direct third party reimbursement for nurses.

Collaborative Practice

Setting up a group practice with one or more nurses involves the same steps one would follow as a solo practitioner except that you may elect to file the necessary legal documents to form a partnership (14).

Interdisciplinary group practice is more complex in some respects and simpler in others. If you are joining the practice of another provider, you will enjoy the advantages of moving into an established office with a caseload already in place. In group practice, financial commitments can vary widely. You may be asked to contribute to operating costs at a percentage based on income generated, at a fixed rate, or at a level allowing you to "buy into" the practice. If you become a salaried employee of a group, your role in decision making will be significantly different than if you are a partner. That is an important distinction to make when considering the various alternatives for financial arrangements. It is impossible to become an owner or shareholder in an incorporated practice or enter into a business partnership. Since regulations vary from state to state with regard to interdisciplinary professional corporations or partnerships, it is best to engage the services of an attorney (15). In 1979, California passed a bill permitting registered nurses to own up to 49% of shares in professional medical corporations (16). Since that time, some other states have followed their example.

You might also choose to enter into a collaborative relationship with other providers whereby you each contribute to overhead expenses but keep separate business accounts, billing procedures, fee schedules, and so on. You then could set up protocols for consultation with the others and they with you on a fee-for-service, reciprocal or gratis arrangement. You and another provider might also wish to consider contracting with each other for services on the basis of a guaranteed income or on a fee-for-service basis. A nurse and a physician might contract for the services of a nutritionist, or a physician might contract for the services of a nurse practitioner/clinical nurse specialist, or vice versa.

Thus, as can be seen, there are a number of interesting arrangements to consider when preparing to set up a collaborative practice (17). Gathering data and assessing each option will enable you to make a decision based on a thorough understanding of the advantages and disadvantages of each. There are also numerous examples in the literature of nurses in collaborative practices as entrepreneurs, exploring and creating new roles and serving new markets (18).

New Models of Entrepreneurial Practice

Several entrepreneurial models for advanced practice have emerged since Lucille Kinlein hung out her shingle. It might be argued that, in some ways, nurses have always found ways to be entrepreneurs, for there are numerous examples such as Jane Hitchcock working independently teaching public health nursing in schools of nursing (19). The advent of advanced practice as clinical nurse specialists and nurse practitioners meant new opportunities for nurse entrepreneurs. Consultation and health education, maternity fitness, home care services for special client groups including persons with AIDS, endstage renal disease, new babies and children with chronic care needs, stress management, nurse managed centers, private case management, and media services are only some of the innovative businesses begun by nurses prepared for advanced practice (18, 21). The term intrapreneurial practice has been applied to nurses organizing as a company to provide nursing services to agencies and institutions or practicing as affiliates of existing hospitals, in community based nursing centers, in independent practice and in private case management (20, 21a). Several resources for nurses considering entrepreneurial roles are included in the bibliography.

Being Employed as a Clinical Nurse Specialist or a Nurse Practitioner

The majority of nurses in advanced practice are employees of physicians, clinics, hospitals, schools, neighborhood and rural health centers, public and private agencies and institutions, and industry (22). As such, they are in an employee-employer relationship and are salaried. The economic aspects of practice as an employee are much less complex than those of the independent practitioner. It is the employer's responsibility to provide office space, equipment, supplies, and so on, while the nurse has to concern her/himself with salary, benefits, malpractice insurance, and the uniforms and equipment which she or he is required to supply. Some employers provide malpractice insurance coverage for their employees, but you may choose to carry your own as well. It is important to keep a record of expenditures that fall under the category of professional expenses in order to receive income tax deductions. With the revised tax laws, it is best to consult a tax expert. Some of these items are listed in Table 10.4.

The nurse employed in a nonprofit rural or neighborhood health clinic or in a voluntary nonprofit agency such as a visiting nurse service

---

Table 10.4 Items that May Qualify for Deductions as Professional Expenses

Uniforms, lab coats, special shoes, stockings
Examination and other equipment
Professional licensure and certification fees and membership dues
Subscription costs for professional journals and newsletters
Malpractice insurance
Costs of continuing education courses, conferences, seminars
Travel to professional meetings, conferences, and travel to and from place of employment for business purposes (meetings, home visits) excluding travel between work and home
Typing, word processing, photocopying, secretarial costs and supplies for professional publication which you must pay for such as envelopes, paper, labels, tape, printer cartridges, floppy diskettes, reproduction of photographs, grapic art
Per diem costs for attendance at meetings, conferences, continuing education
Professional gifts and entertaining
Books, calculated on a time depreciation basis
Purchase of a typewriter, computer, camera, tape recorder, fax machine, answering machine, or other equipment used for business — calculated on a depreciation basis
Child care expenses associated with work
Postage
Professional phone calls
Tuition for credit courses
Travel for consultation or meetings with other providers or related to professional publication
Printing costs for business cards and resumes, stationery, rubber stamps, name pins
Disposables such as batteries or ear cones for otoscope, penlight
Home office

---

may be more involved in the financial aspects of the agency than the employee of a hospital or industry because positions may be dependent upon soft monies or, in part, upon contributions or donations. Part of the job, then, may involve grant writing or public relations work to generate support for the ongoing operation of the service. Employees of agencies seeking rural health clinic status may have to participate in a community assessment in order to demonstrate why the application should be considered.

Some employers may look at productivity for an index of the cost effectiveness of nurses' services. Such evaluations must consider more than the size of the caseload or number of patient visits (23, 24) and should include a multipractice factor analysis of cost effectiveness to provide data to support the need for positions and for nurses as members of the health care team.

Third Party Reimbursement

Several attempts to bring about change in reimbursement policies to nurses have been made, the earliest in 1948 (25), and some of these efforts have been successful and will be described here. However, present reimbursement schemes in many states still not only preclude third party reimbursement for nurses and other non-physician providers, but also limit access for clients who are unable to pay out-of-pocket. Thus, many consumers are not able to have direct access to nursing services. The present system is based on the assumption that the physician is the appropriate provider for the client's needs (26), or at least the gatekeeper for the system.

Recognizing the importance of developing new models for reimbursement for providers, Congress, in the Social Security Amendments of 1972 (P.L. 92-603), authorized experiments and demonstration projects focused on methods and amounts of reimbursement for services performed by independent providers. Thus the Physician Extender Reimbursement Study was launched (27). While nurses may react unfavorably to being classified as "physician extenders," the concept of independent reimbursement is critical.

On numerous occasions, Senator Inouye of Hawaii has introduced bills to amend the Social Security Act to allow for direct reimbursement for nursing services under Medicaid and Medicare. Early versions were directed at reimbursing certified psychiatric nurses with master's degrees who worked in community mental health programs (28). In later bills sponsored by Senator Inouye, proposals were made to allow direct reimbursement of registered nurses and nurse-midwives under Medicare and Medicaid (29, 30).

By 1979, sixteen states had authorized payment for nurse-midwives under Medicaid (31). In that year, a bill was proposed by Representative Barbara Mikulski of Maryland to allow Medicaid reimbursement for nurse-midwives (32). The Department of Defense had previously adopted a policy for direct payment for nurse-midwives through CHAMPUS, its program for the health care of dependents (31). In 1982, direct reimbursement for nurse-midwives was authorized through Medicaid (33). Since that time, the federal government has allowed states to administer Medicaid within broad general guidelines. Often this means only policy change for nurses to get direct reimbursement (34).

In 1980, Maryland became the first state to provide for direct reimbursement for nurses and other non-physician providers through all health insurance (35). Maryland had previously passed bills allowing reimbursement for nurse-midwives and nurse practitioners (36, 37, 38).

The Rural Health Clinic Services (RHCS) Act of 1977 (P.L. 95-210) authorizes Medicare and Medicaid payments to qualified rural health clinics for the services of nurse practitioners (39). Clinics must apply to become certified in order to be eligible for reimbursement. In 1988, changes in the Act rekindled interest in use of its provisions to assist rural hospitals and health clinics (40), and in the Omnibus Budget Reconciliation Act of 1989, new RHCS provisions enhanced its potential for advanced practitioners (41).

By 1993, 38 states had passed legislation recognizing some form of third-party reimbursement for nurses' services, and other states were considering similar bills. Some states which have passed legislation specify reimbursement for nurse practitioners, some for nurse-midwives, and some for a variety of nurses in advanced practice positions (42).

Additionally, a number of states have recognized third-party reimbursement for nurses under Medicaid as provided in a 1990 federal law. In 1989, legislation was passed by Congress to allow Medicare reimbursement for nurse practitioner care in long-term care, and bills have been introduced to extend Medicare and Medicaid reimbursement in other settings and for other advanced practice nurses (43). Third-party reimbursement through Blue Cross/Blue Shield and private insurance carriers is also available to nurses in some states (44). And in 37 states, some advanced practice nurses in specified categories are receiving direct reimbursement from private insurance companies, although in many states no legislative authority exists as yet (42). In fact, private insurers can establish their own policies, so legislative change is often not necessary.

In 1987, the Federal Employees Health Care Freedom of Choice Act was introduced to Congress and passed by it. This bill mandates direct third party reimbursement to nurses, nurse practitioners, nurse-midwives, and several other non-physician health care providers under the Federal Employees Health Benefits Program. This bill has important implications for nurses in advanced practice (46, 47).

It seems evident that if nurses are to achieve full recognition under third party reimbursement plans, both federal and private, we must be politically active. Jennings (48) suggests we might form political action partnerships with groups such as the American Association of Retired Persons. We must be in the forefront of health policy decision-making and utilize the power inherent in the numbers of health care providers we represent when national health insurance or similar plans are proposed. To paraphrase Jennings, we must be recognized as essential providers of care (48). If we are not strong participants in forming national health policy, others will do it for us.

Advanced Practitioners: Benefits and Cost Effectiveness of Their Practice

In a compelling article, Safriet argues that advanced practice nurses are cost-effective, deliver high quality care to clients who are very needy, and that limitations on scope of practice, third-part reimbursement and prescription writing privileges should be eliminated. Her thorough review of these issues provides a useful tool for several purposes: legislative and policy change at the state level; health care reform at the state and federal level; negotiating positions in employing agencies, institutions, and group practices; and in documenting the cost effectiveness and benefits of advanced practice nurses (49).

Numerous models have been proposed and tested for assessing the cost-effectiveness and benefits of nurses in a variety of advanced practice roles (50, 51, 52, 53, 54). Some of these have clinical utility as part of quality improvement programs. They also help nurses to assess how they spend their time, the revenues they generate for the agency or practice, and how they might alter their activities to prevent burnout. Incorporating such data collection as part of roles in advanced practice will help to assure that advanced practitioners are not forgotten in health care reform.

Salaries and Employment of Nurses in Advanced Practice

Salary and employment characteristics of nurses in advanced practice are useful in negotiating for a position and, in particular, in instituting an advanced practice role in an agency, institution or practice where there has not been an advanced practitioner before. There are several sources of data on such issues. The *American Journal of Nursing* has an annual report on nursing salaries and benefits. Several specialty organizations and state nurse practitioner groups have conducted and published salary surveys. The American Nurses Association and its Council of Nurses in Advanced Practice collects data on characteristics of employment of nurses in advanced practice roles. Several interdisciplinary organizations and publications also conduct salary surveys.

Some of the recent surveys are interesting to set a context for advanced practice nurses. A survey of salaries for professionals in family planning revealed that setting for practice, region of the country, and subspecialties are more important salary determinants than are advanced degrees (55). One study of nurse practitioner salaries and benefits revealed a range of less than $15,000 to more than $40,000 and a wide array of benefits (56). In the 1992 *American Journal of Nursing* survey, nurse practitioner salaries were lower than those of clinical nurse specialists in hospitals, but higher in medical schools and the same in medical centers (57). As the authors of one study suggest, nurse practitioners (and other nurses in advanced practice) should learn to negotiate for salary and benefits commensurate with the value of their services (56).

Marketing

It is clear that other health care professionals are marketing their services to the public. If we are to succeed in a competitive health care arena, we must learn to market ourselves. Strategies can include hosting a talk show on health care issues, writing a column or an editorial for a local newspaper, advertisements, news releases, fact sheets, brochures, newsletters for consumers, direct mailings, conducting marketing surveys (see Chapter 12), personal interviews in the media, speeches to lay groups, and developing a profile of providers who might be potential competitors as well as referents (58, 59). Marketing includes selling ourselves to other health care providers as well as to the public. Our relationships with clients will demonstrate what we have to offer. There are numerous resources in the literature on marketing strategies, and there are classes and courses on the subject offered at colleges, universities, and adult education programs (59).

Summary

It is clear that nursing is at an economic crossroad. We can content ourselves with being cogs in the giant economic machine of our health care system or we can seize the power that is rightfully ours as the largest group of professional providers.

If we are to be creators of policy for health care, it is important to strengthen our position by researching the costs of nursing services delivered through nursing models, educating the public as to the value of nursing services, soliciting consumer advocacy for nurses, and gaining control of our practice within our work settings (60).

Most of all, to quote Alford, we must "no longer stand in the shadow of medicine but must come out into the light, indeed into the glare, of center stage and be recognized for [our] unique contribution to health care" (60).

REFERENCES

1. Rew, L. (1988). AFFIRM the role of clinical specialist in private practice. Clinical Nurse Specialist 2(1):39-43. 1.
2. Edmunds, M. (1980). Financial planning for independent practice. The Nurse Practitioner 5:35-36, 38.
3. Simms, E. (1977). Preparation for independent practice. Nursing Outlook 25:114-118.
4. Dalton, J.B. (1985). Guide to private practice office planning. The Nurse Practitioner 10(5):43-44, 47, 56.
5. Jacox, A.K. & Norris, C.M. (Eds.) (1977). Organizing for Independent Nursing Practice. New York: Appleton-Century-Crofts. p. 127.
6. Kinlein, M.L. (1977). Independent Nursing Practice with Clients. Philadelphia: J.B. Lippincott. p. 37.
7. McShane, N.G. & Smith, E.M. (1978). Starting a private practice in mental health nursing. American Journal of Nursing 78:2068-2070.
8. RN fights for title in phone directory. (1981). American Journal of Nursing 81:265.
9. Pearson, L.J. (1986). Nancy Dirubbo: Fighting for the rights of NPs in private practice. The Nurse Practitioner 11(9):52, 57-58, 62.
10. Nichols, J.S. & Nichols, R.E. (1990). How to start a practice on a shoestring. Journal of American Academy of Nurse Practitioners 2(3):129-131.
11. Koltz, C.J. (1979). Private Practice in Nursing. Germantown, MD: Aspen. p. 145.
12. Jacox, A.K. & Norris, C.M., op.cit., pp. 128-129.
13. Kinlein, M.C., op.cit., p. 44.
14. Thomas, C. (1986). How to join and participate in a medical corporation. The Nurse Practitioner 11(9):64, 67, 71.

15. Jacox, A.K. & Norris, C.M. op. cit., pp. 144-145.
16. California RNs can now own shares in joint RN-MD professional practices. (1979). American Journal of Nursing 79:2074.
17. Wille, R. & Frederickson, K.C. (1981). Establishing a group private practice in nursing. Nursing Outlook 29:522-524.
18. Clark, L. & Quinn, J. (1988). The new entrepreneurs. Nursing and Health Care 9(1):7-15.
19. Kaufman, M., Hawkins, J.W., Higgins, L.P. & Friedman, A.H. (1988). Dictionary of American Nursing Biography. New York: Greenwood Press.
20. American Nurses Association. (1987). The nursing center: Concept and design. Kansas City, MO: ANA.
21. Wallace, B. Nurses move outside traditional roles. NAACOG Newsletter, June, 1987.
21a. Boyer, D.C. & Martinson, D.J. (1990). Intrapreneurial group practice. Nursing & Health Care II(1):29-32.
22. Facts about Nursing 86-87. (1987). Kansas City, MO: American Nurses' Association.
23. Mahoney, D.F. (1988). An economic analysis of the nurse practitioner role. The Nurse Practitioner 13(3):44-45, 48-50, 52.
24. Lockhart, C.A. (1985). Nursing's future in a shrinking health care system. In: G.E. Sorenson (Ed.): The Economics of Health Care and Nursing. Kansas City, MO: American Academy of Nursing. pp. 19-29.
25. Jennings, C.P. (1977). Third party reimbursement and the nurse practitioner. The Nurse Practitioner 2:11-13.
26. Caraher, M.T. (1988). The importance of third-party reimbursement for NPs. The Nurse Practitioner 13(4):50, 52, 54.
27. Morris, S.B. & Smith, D.B. (1976). The Physician Extender Reimbursement Study. The Diffusion of Physician Extenders (Working Paper No. 1). Washington, DC: U.S. Social Security Administration, Office of Research and Statistics.
28. New senate bill provides Medicare and Medicaid reimbursement systems for psychiatric nursing. (1976). American Journal of Nursing 76:1220-1221.
29. Inouye bill would reimburse RNs directly under Medicare/Medi-

caid. (1977). American Journal of Nursing 77:349.
30. Inouye bill S. 1702 proposes payment to nurse-midwives under Medicaid/Medicare. (1977). American Journal of Nursing 77:1241, 1244.
31. ANA backs direct reimbursement to nurse-midwives under Medicare. (1979). American Journal of Nursing 79:2070.
32. Nurse-midwife payments OKed with Medicare-Medicaid bill. (1981). American Journal of Nursing 81:338, 448, 466.
33. Nurse-midwives win direct reimbursement under Medicaid. (1982). American Journal of Nursing 82:1335.
34. Pearson, L.J. (1990). The issue of third-party reimbursement — advice for nurse practitioners from a national expert. The Nurse Practitioner 15(3):46-47.
35. Maryland is first state to require third-party payment for nurses. (1980). American Journal of Nursing 80:7.
36. CNM services are reimbursable in Maryland. (1978). American Journal of Nursing 78:1143-1178.
37. Griffith, H.M. (1982). Strategies for direct third-party reimbursement for nurses. American Journal of Nursing 82:408-411.
38. Goldwater, M. (1982). From a legislator: Views on third-party reimbursement for nurses. American Journal of Nursing 82:411-414.
39. Rural Health Clinic Services. (1979). Hyattsville, MD: Department of Health, Education, and Welfare. p. 1.
40. Rural Health Clinics Act offers revenue benefits. (1988) The Nurse Practitioner 13(8):64, 66.
41. Wasem, C. (1990). The Rural Health Clinic Services Act: A sleeping giant of reimbursement. Journal of the Aemrican Academy of Nurse Practitioners 2(2):85-87.
42. Pearson, L.J. (1993). 1992-93 update: How each state stands on legislative issues affecting advanced nursing practice. The Nurse Practitioner 18(1):25.
43. Towers, J. (1992). The status of Medicare reimbursement for nurse practitioners. Journal of the American Academy of Nurse Practitioners 4(3):129-130.
44. Pearson, L.J. (1993). op cit.

45. Pearson, L.J. (1993, op cit.
46. Knox, J.T. (1988). Direct reimbursement to nurse practitioners: The importance of the Federal Employees Health Care Freedom of Choice Act (H.R. 382). The Nurse Practitioner 13(11):52-53.
47. Stallmeyer, J. (1986). Direct reimbursement for NPs under FEHBP. The Nurse Practitioner 11(6):14,16.
48. Jennings, C.P. (1979). Nursing's case for third party reimbursement. American Jurnal of Nursing 79:111-114.
49. Safriet, B.J. (1992). Health care dollars and regulatory sense: The role of advanced practice nursing. Yale Journal on Regulation 9:417-488.
50. Gift, A.G. (1992). Determining CNS cost effectiveness. Clinical Nurse Specialist 6(2):89.
51. McGrath, S. (1990). The cost-effectiveness of nurse practitioners. The Nurse Practitioner 15(7):40-42.
52. Gardner, D. (1992). The CNS as a cost manager. Clinical Nurse Specialist 6(2):112-116.
53. Edwardson, S.R. (1992). Costs and benefits of clinical nurse specialists. Clinical Nurse Specialist 6(3):163-167.
54. Kearnes, D.R. (1992). A productivity tool to evaluate NP practice: Monitoring clinical time spent in reimbursable patient-related activities. The Nurse Practitioner 17(4):50; 52; 55.
55. 1992 salary survey results. Contraceptive Technology Update, supplement. 1992. 1-10.
56. Rogers, B., Sweeting, S. & Davis, B. (1989). Employment and salary characteristics of nurse practitioners. The Nurse Practitioner 14(9):56; 59-60; 63; 66.
57. Brider, P. (1992). Salary gains slow as more RNs seek full-time benefits. American Journal of Nursing 92(3):34-40.
58. Pearson, L.J. (1986). Jo Ann Woodward: Opening channels of communication: Marketing the NP role. The Nurse Practitioner 11(11):55,59-60,62.
59. Gardner, K.L. & Weinrauch, D.(1988). Marketing strategies for nurse entrepreneurs. The Nurse Practitioner 13(5):46, 48-49.
60. Alford, D.M. (1979). Cost-effective empirical model of an ambulatory nursing practice. In: Nursing's Influence on Health

Policy for the Eighties. Kansas City, MO: American Academy of Nursing. pp. 40-44.

BIBLIOGRAPHY

Change from Within: Nurse Intrapreneurs as Health Care Innovators. 1990.*
Earn What You're Worth: A Nurse's Guide to Better Compensation. 1989.*
The Nurse Entrepreneur: A Reference Manual for Business Design. 1989.*
Gardner, K.L. & Weinrauch, D. (1988). Marketing strategies for nurse entrepreneurs. The Nurse Practitioner 13(5):46-49.
New Organizational Models and Financial Arrangements for Nursing Services. 1986.*
Nurse Entrepreneur Handbook, 1990. Ohio Nurses Association, 4000 East Main Street, Columbus, Ohio 43213-2983.
Nurse in Private Practice: Characteristics, Organizational Arrangements and Reimbursement Policy. 1988.*
Rauen, K., Sperry, C. & Miller, J. (1988). The Nurse Intrapreneur: Opportunities and Benefits for Nursing. Philadelphia: Lippincott.
Vogel, G. & Doleysh, N. (1988). Entrepreneuring: A Nurse's Guide to Starting a Business. New York: National League for Nursing.

---

*Publications available from American Nurses Publishing, American Nurses Association, 600 Maryland Avenue SW, Suite 100 West, Washington, DC 20024-2571.

11
Mentorship

Introduction

Although mentoring is an ancient concept, it is only recently that nursing leaders have actively explored the benefits of mentorship to the profession. Every practitioner or clinician needs to make an informed choice about whether to enter into a mentoring relationship and understand what the effects of that decision may have on his or her career development. This chapter clarifies some of the misconceptions surrounding mentorship and explores the advantages and drawbacks of being a mentor or mentee. The developmental stages of a mentoring relationship, the desired characteristics of a mentor and a mentee, and alternatives to mentoring are also presented.

What Mentorship Is

The concept of the mentor has its origins in Greek mythology. Athena, goddess of wisdom, disguised herself as Mentor, a wise old nobleman, in order to act as the self-appointed guardian to Telemachus, the son of Ulysses, during Ulysses' 20-year absence from home during the Trojan wars. Mentor acted as protector, advisor, and guide to Telemachus. It is ironic to note that the first mentor was a woman whose role was to guide and facilitate the career development of a young man. Until the women's movement of the sixties, writers paid little attention to the role of women as mentors or mentees.

Levinson (1), in *The Seasons of a Man's Life,* expands upon the roles of protector, advisor, and guide, and identifies additional mentor sub-roles: teacher, sponsor, host, counselor, and exemplar. In the role of teacher, the mentor helps to develop the mentee's intellectual and career-related skills. As sponsor, the mentor uses his or her reputation and network of personal contacts to facilitate the mentee's entry into the work place in order to promote more rapid career advancement. As host and guide, the mentor introduces the mentee into the informal social network or "locker room" where many of the influential career decisions are made. Advice, guidance, moral support, and nurturance comprise the counselor sub-role. As exemplar, the mentor provides a standard of excellence which the mentee can aspire to or surpass.

A mentor, however, is not just a teacher or a sponsor or a role model. A mentor is a combination of all of the sub-roles which comprise a true mentorship: mentorship is greater than the sum of its parts. It is an intense, sustained, long-term relationship between a novice and a recognized expert in a given discipline (2). Mentorship does not happen by accident. It is the result of a conscious choice by both parties. The mentor is involved with the mentee in both a cognitive and an affective relationship of trust, preference, and mutuality (3). Mentorship is a careful, nurturing support system essential to the novice's professional development, career success, and satisfaction.

Many have said that a career without a mentor is doomed to failure: a mentor is necessary and essential to career success. May, Meleis, and Winstead-Fry (3) believe that "mentorship and sponsorship are essential for the scholarly development of nurses and for the integration of the scholarly role in the self." They go on to say that "aspirations to scholarliness are not innate but learned; such aspirations are developed in some novices and enhanced in others through mentorship and sponsorship."

There are many books and articles that advise young professionals to identify a mentor and to get one as soon as possible. A mentor is portrayed as the means to get to the top of the career ladder in the most direct and efficacious manner. Sheehy (4) states that, virtually without exception, the successful women she has studied have been nurtured by a mentor. Henning and Jardim, in their popular best seller, *The Managerial Woman* (5), concluded that career success depends upon a mentoring relationship with one's boss or superior. Kanter, in *Men and Women of the Corporation* (6), reinforced Sheehy and Henning's findings and observed that the sponsorship of high level, powerful "rabbis" or "godfathers" largely determines who gets ahead. It would seem then that in order to insure career success every nurse should find a powerful "godmother" or "godfather."

Benefits to the Mentor

To be sure, there can be definite advantages for both parties involved in a mentoring relationship. Erikson (7) states that the prime developmental task of the mid-career years is generativity versus stagnation. Mentorship is one way of countering mid-career obsolescence and boredom. There is a sense of personal satisfaction and pride gained from seeing a colleague one has nurtured gain success and career satisfaction. In Maslow's (8) terms, mentorship may be viewed as the ultimate self-actualization: feeling good enough about one's self and one's achievements to generously and selflessly help another reach his or her potential. The mentoring relationship may actually help the mentee surpass the accomplishments of the mentor and achieve greater fame and recognition.

On a more practical level, a mentor can gain more control over his or her work environment by spending time on those activities which require particular expertise and by delegating other tasks to the mentee who is learning the skills required in the early stages of career development. A mentor's reputation can also be enhanced by a "following" of mentees who serve as testimony to the mentor. This enhancement of the mentor's reputation can sometimes lead to lucrative offers to serve as a consultant, conduct workshops, or become part of other professional endeavors.

Benefits to the Mentee

Phillips-Jones (9), Kram (10), and Fowler (11), among others, have lauded the benefits of having a mentor because it can lead to:

- more rapid career advancement
- greater knowledge of the intricacies of a given system or organization
- ease of acceptance into the socio-political network
- higher publication rates
- publication in more prestigious journals
- more research funding
- choice committee assignments

Mentorship can also increase personal satisfaction and self-esteem by having an esteemed and respected colleague pay personal attention to a young, promising novice.

Disadvantages of the Mentoring Relationship

Before jumping on the mentoring bandwagon, let us look at the other side of the issue. In the clinical setting particularly, a potential mentor may have an actual or perceived work overload and may feel that a mentee would contribute to that overload rather than help redistribute time and energy in a more advantageous manner. If a mentor does not enter into the mentoring relationship willingly and with a positive attitude, then neither party will benefit from the mentorship arrangement in the long run.

Blotnick (12) tracked 3,000 mentor-protege pairs over a three-year period and found that two-thirds of the pairs ended up disenchanted with their relationships. Because the mentoring relationship is an intense one, it is subject to the same stressors and problems as a relationship between spouses. Just as tension in a marriage can lead to dissatisfaction and divorce, tension in a mentoring relationship can lead to an unhappy parting.

A mentoring relationship may be particularly at risk if the mentor and mentee pair are also boss and subordinate. Blotnick (12) found that in cases of conflict in these pairs, 40 percent of the mentors fired the mentee. The mentor got tired of the constant tension and removed its perceived source.

May, Meleis, and Winstead-Fry (3) identify other potential problems inherent in the mentoring relationship: dependence, exploitation, and lack of individuation. Because mentoring is a nurturing relationship, a mentor may become too "motherly" or overprotective with resultant dependency and passivity on the part of the mentee. The mentor may make the career climb too easy for the mentee. This may ultimately be detrimental to the mentee who never learns risk-taking, problem-solving, and conflict-resolution behaviors.

Creativity and independence may be sacrificed for the safe tried-and-tested path. Maintenance of the status quo is not only detrimental to an individual's career, but to the nursing profession as well. Nursing is still struggling with issues of autonomy, assertiveness, and independence. A mentoring relationship between two female nurses can be at high risk for the dependence dilemma.

In addition to a balance between independence-dependence, a balance must exist between cooperation and competition in the mentorship. Over-competitiveness or extreme cooperation by either party can result in one person being overpowered and exploited by the other. An example of this situation is the well-known "Queen Bee' syndrome. The "Queen" cannot tolerate criticism, collaboration, conflicting ideas, or sharing the praise for joint endeavors, all of which are the primary behaviors desired in a good mentor (13). The mentee may develop into a drone whose role is to stroke the ego of the mentor to the detriment of establishing his or her own individual career identity.

Choice of Mentor

Awareness of the potential pitfalls of a mentoring relationship should not necessarily steer you away from one, but should instead help you make careful choices. The choice of a mentor is a crucial one that requires careful consideration and exploration before a formal arrangement is established. The mentor is a person with whom you will work closely for a number of years. For starters, you should enjoy this person's company and like spending time with him or her.

If at all possible, you should avoid having your direct supervisor as your mentor. Issues of subservience, on-the-job conflict, complaints of favoritism by other colleagues, and the possibility of being fired are mitigated if you are not working directly under your mentor. Also avoid choosing a close personal friend, but choose instead a respected, professional colleague with whom you do not have a social relationship. Although a mentoring relationship is a close one, it is a professional association and issues of friendship complicate it.

View the mentoring relationship as a long-term one, but also as a temporary one. It is not a life-long commitment. Establish a three-year contract with explicit goals and objectives to be mutually reviewed on an ongoing basis. If the relationship is not meeting desired goals, it needs to be altered or terminated before irremediable differences occur. Mentoring, or a given mentor, may be beneficial at one stage of your career but not at others. In order for mentoring to be successful, both parties must believe it is meeting agreed-upon objectives. This can only be ascertained by frank ongoing discussions. It goes without saying that your choice of mentor should be someone with whom you believe you can freely communicate.

A review of the mentoring research yields some additional tips which might be useful in the choice of a mentor. You must select a person in whom you have trust and confidence. This person must have the ability to motivate you to do your very best. The potential mentor must be respected in the area of your particular interest and have proven leadership ability. The mentor must have a great deal of confidence in his or her own abilities and must be happy with his or her own career success.

It is also recommended that, ideally, the mentor be eight to 15 years older than you are. This age difference provides a one-half generational split and helps to avoid parenting or peer dilemmas. There is no general consensus as to whether a same-sex person makes a better mentor than a person of the opposite sex. It may be easier for a mentee to identify with a person of the same sex, but over-identification may then become an issue. Mixed pairs, on the other hand, may have to deal with sexual issues and patronage. The best advice is to choose the person, regardless of sex, who is most compatible with you and can best help you achieve your career goals.

Finding a suitable mentor is only half of the equation. Are you a suitable mentee? You must be ready and willing to learn, dream, and invest yourself and your time in an intensive, goal-directed relationship. You need to view yourself as upwardly mobile and embarking on a long-term career path with specific goals. If this is you — go to it and seek a compatible mentor.

Stages of the Mentoring Relationship

Like any relationship, mentoring has developmental stages. These stages parallel career developmental tasks. Recognition of the stages of mentoring can help both parties plan appropriate activities and deal with potential crises inherent in each stage. The first of the mentoring relationship stages may be called the *invitational stage*. This is analogous to the honeymoon stage of social relationships or group behavior. Both parties display their best behaviors while carefully testing out their visions of the relationship.

The globally positive feelings of the relationship are soon replaced by fears about how the relationship will actually work out and by the realization that much hard work is involved. The pendulum swings from positive feelings to uneasy or negative ones. This stage has been referred to as the questioning stage. This is an opportune time to clarify initial impressions and solidify the parameters of the working relationship.

The questioning stage is followed by, hopefully, the longest phase of the relationship, the *informational stage* or *working stage*. However, if earlier conflicts are not resolved, the relationship will continually return to the questioning stage and energy will be expended in conflict rather than in output. The working stage is the time when the mentee actually "learns the ropes," discovers the political networks and power sources, and learns the game plan and how to master it. The mentee should be involved in concrete activities such as special projects, committee work, research, and publication under the guidance of the mentor.

As with all relationships, the final stage is *termination* (14). Termination always has both positive and negative feelings associated with it. A mentorship may terminate before the time of the predetermined contract if there is conflict, changing career interests on the part of either or both parties, or circumstantial factors such as a move to another location. The relationship may also terminate because it is successful and has achieved the desired outcome. The mentee is ready to move on and assume the responsibilities of the next phase of career development. Termination should not just happen abruptly, but should be planned and discussed, as were the other phases. An unresolved termination detracts from career success in the next phases of the career ladder. Wheatley and Hirsh (15) give a detailed account of some of the emotional issues involved in the termination phase and offer concrete suggestions for dealing with these issues.

Alternatives to Mentoring

If mentoring is not for you, or a suitable mentor is not available, there are alternatives to explore. One avenue is having multiple mentors as opposed to an intensive relationship with a single mentor. This situation gives you the opportunity to seek and receive advice from several sources and avoids the potential pitfalls of an exclusive relationship.

Publications which give concrete, career-related information can serve as "paper mentors." Examples of paper mentors are given at the end of this chapter. Career interest subgroups of professional nursing organization can also provide some of the services a mentor offers, such as the guidance and advice of experts in the field.

Networks can also serves as mentors. Networks consist of persons who know about the system, have achieved some measure of career success, and meet on a formal or informal basis. Networks help new professionals establish valuable contacts and often serve as support groups. Networking may actually produce a sponsor or mentor or at least put you in contact with those in a position to recognize and reward good performance and make crucial recommendations (16).

Conclusion

Mentorship can play a vital role in the career development of the nurse practitioner or clinician if that individual makes careful, informed decisions and choices. A mentoring relationship requires forethought and planning. Mentorship offers an opportunity to both mentors and mentees to embark on a mutually satisfying contractual relationship with beneficial career rewards.

REFERENCES

1. Levinson, D.J. (1978). The Seasons of a Man's Life. New York: Knopf.
2. Schmidt, J.A. & Wolf, J.S. (1980). The master partnership: Discovery of professionalism. National Association of Student Personnel Administrators Journal 17:45-51.
3. May, K., Meleis, A. & Winstead-Fry, P. (1982). Mentorship for scholarship: Opportunities and dilemmas. Nursing Outlook 30(1):22-28.
4. Sheehy, G. (1976). The mentor connection and the secret link in the successful woman's life. New York 8:33-39.
5. Henning, M. & Jardim, A. (1977). The Managerial Woman. New York: Anchor Press/Doubleday.
6. Kanter, R.M. (1977). Men and Women of the Corporation. New York: Basic Books.
7. Erikson, E. (1963). Childhood and Society. New York: W.W. Norton.
8. Maslow, A.H. (1968). Toward a Psychology of Being. 2nd. ed. New York: Van Nostrand Reinhold.
9. Phillips-Jones, L. (1982). Mentor and Proteges: How to Establish, Strengthen and Get the Most from a Mentor/ Protege Relationship. New York: Arbor House.
10. Kram, K. (1984). Mentoring at Work: Developmental Relation-

ships in Organizational Life. New York: Scotts Foresman.
11. Fowler, D.L. (1986). Mentoring relationships and the perceived quality of the academic work environment. In: P. Farrant (Ed.), Strategies and Attitudes. Women in Educational Administration. Washington, DC: National Association for Women Deans, Administrators, and Counselors (NAWDAC). pp. 77-83.
12. Blotnick, S.R. (1984). With friends like these. Savvy 10:45-52.
13. White, M.D. (1972). The importance of selected nursing activities. Nursing Research 21:4-14.
14. Keele, R.L. & DeLaMare-Schaefer, M. (1984). So what do you do now that you don't have a mentor? Journal of National Association for Women Deans, Administrators, and Counselors, Spring:36-40.
15. Wheatley, M. & Hirsch, M.S. (1984). Five ways to leave your mentor. Ms. Magazine. Sept.:106-108.
16. Barrax, J.D. (1986). A comparative profile of female and male university administrators. In: P. Farrant (Ed.), Strategies and Attitudes. Women in Educational Administration. Washington, DC: National Association for Women Deans, Administrators, and Counselors. pp. 59-64.

PAPER MENTORS

Beck, L. (1989). Mentorships: Benefits and effects on career development. Gifted Child Quarterly 33(1):23-28.
Boyle, C. & James, S. (1990). Nurses as leaders: How are we doing? Nursing Administration Quarterly 15:44-48.
Brito, H. (1992). Nurses in action: An innovative approach to mentoring. Journal of Nursing Administration 22:23-28.
Fields, W.L. (1991). Mentoring in nursing: A historical approach. Nursing Outlook 39(6):257-261.
Haas, S.A. (1992). Coaching. Developing key players. Journal of Nursing Administration 22:54-58.
Kirk, E.k & Reichart, G. (1992). The mentoring relationship: What makes it work? Imprint 39:20-22.

Mateo, M.A. (1992). Publication skill development in nurses. Journal of Nursing Administration 22:64-66.

Miller, F.A. (1992). Leadership strategies for professional development. Journal of the National Black Nurses Association 5:54-60.

Prestholdt, C. (1990). Modern mentoring: Strategies for developing contemporary nursing leadership. Nursing Administration Quarterly 15:20-27.

12

Community Assessment

Introduction

Since the inception of the first clinical specialist program in 1954 and the first nurse practitioner program in 1965, nurses with advanced preparation have served both the "haves" and "have nots" in the health care delivery system. Stating that "nursing is not second class medicine but first class health care" (1), Loretta Ford went on to challenge nurses to demonstrate their value in industrial settings and with the poor and the underserved. The American Nurses Association, in its 1980 social policy statement on nursing, cites identifying populations at risk as one of the functions of nursing specialists (2). And as early as 1971, the report to the Secretary of the Department of Health, Education and Welfare prepared by the Secretary's Committee to Study Extended Roles for Nurses called "assessing community resources and needs for health care" one of the responsibilities of nurses with advanced preparation (3).

Community assessment is one type of market survey for identifying groups of inadequately served clients that nurses might appropriately serve.

The concept of nursing's involvement in community assessment is not unique to the roles of nurses today. In the early decades of this century, Lillian Wald observed the needs of the tenement dwellers in New York City and took steps to meet those needs through expanding the role of public health nurses and establishing the Henry Street Settlement (4). She also saw a need for a stronger commitment to the health and welfare of the children of this country and, in so doing, was instrumental in founding the Children's Bureau in 1912 (5). In 1925, Mary Breckinridge, recognizing the unmet needs of children and their families in the Kentucky mountains, founded the Frontier Nursing Service (6). And, although not prepared as a nurse, Jane Addams recognized the need for nursing care for families in the neighborhood surrounding Hull House in the Chicago of the late nineteenth and early twentieth centuries. When the Visiting Nurse Association of Chicago was founded, Hull House was chosen as a site for one of its district substations (7).

The Nurse's Role in Identifying Underserved Groups

Thus, our heritage as providers of health care to outcast groups is as old as nursing and marks us a providers who are sensitive and responsive to the changing needs of our clients. Community assessment is a consequence of the evolving roles of nurses as practitioners responsible for the health care of individuals within a community.

The focus of practice for a nurse should extend beyond the confines of her/his own caseload or immediate setting. Utilizing strategies for community assessment, the nurse engaged in an advanced practice role can identify groups ignored or alienated by traditional means of health care delivery. "Primary health care nurses seek out individuals and groups in need, work with others to uncover poor health conditions, and work with the community at large to bring about needed change" (8).

There are three instances where conducting a community assessment constitutes part of the role of the nurse practitioner or clinical nurse specialist: 1) as part of an already existing agency to ascertain that the providers are meeting the needs of those they serve; 2) prior to creating a new practice or service; and 3) as an attempt to expand services or reach out to a changing community.

Who are the groups toward whom nurses might turn their attention in doing a community assessment? Milio (9) identifies these as the poor, those who live in less than desirable locations, ethnic and racial minorities, women, and the aged. These people "lack access to social resources compared to those in the more dominant race, sex, age, income, or geographical groupings." To these we can add the homeless and persons with AIDS. Frontier areas have recently been designated as less than six persons per square mile and with lower health status than other rural citizens. These areas offer a special challenge and opportunity to advanced practitioners (10). Developing the role of the clinical nurse specialist with Native Americans is another example of an underserved group on whom advanced practitioners might focus (11).

Target groups for health and wellness care within the scope of nursing management might include workers, senior citizens, and members of unions (12). Assessments for potential client groups might take place in union halls, retirement housing complexes, senior citizen centers, day care centers, the work place, social organizations, schools, and among consumers, self-help groups, and residents of rural areas.

Conducting a Community Assessment

When making as assessment, all available data should be used in order to get as complete and accurate a picture as possible. To do this within a community, a number of methods may be employed. These include observation, interviews, surveys, use of demographic data, and visits to official agencies such as the Health System Agencies, the Area Health Education Center if one exists, the local health department, and community agencies including the Visiting Nurse Service, senior citizen centers, schools, churches, and the Red Cross chapter (13).

Prior to collecting data, formulate a plan for the assessment. Prepare a purpose and objectives. It is important to be clear about what you wish to find out before you approach individuals or agencies for assistance. Are you planning for an independent practice and assessing for potential clients? Is your agency seeking rural health clinic status? Are you or your agency applying for extramural funding? Does your agency wish to ascertain the needs of the surrounding community, their desire for new services, or reaffirm its role in the community? The cost of doing an assessment must be considered. Will you pay for it as an independent practitioner? Is your agency prepared to cover costs? Can private or public sources be tapped? Computer resources make data collecting, organizing, and managing easier (14).

List all the possible sources of data you require and plan strategies for data collection. The local Health Systems Agency has a wealth of data about the area it serves. Town, county, and state census data can be helpful. Data maintained by schools, courts, police departments, voluntary health-related agencies, community organizations, commercial health-related groups such as Weight Watchers, Diet Workshop, social and fraternal groups, churches, synagogues, as well as those agencies and institutions responsible for direct delivery of health care should not be overlooked if they can contribute information for the assessment (15). "Key informants" are important sources. These may include local housing inspectors, school nurses, public health and parish nurses, welfare and social workers, consumers, members of the local health board, town officials, state senators and representatives, and directors of such groups as Alcoholics Anonymous (15).

An up-to-date map is useful if your assessment covers a geographic area of consequence. Utilize contacts to gain access to those whom you hope to serve if you need their input. For example, you may wish to survey the health needs of all adults over 60 years of age living in a particular town, county, or demarcated area within a city. Utilizing census data, you can estimate the number of such persons and where they reside. To have access to them, unless you are willing to make door to door visits, you next need to find out if and where they congregate. Is there a senior citizen's center in the area? Or a parish church with a large proportion of elders? Since Visiting Nurse or public health nursing services exist in most areas, meet with these providers, explain your purpose, and elicit help.

If your target population consists of working persons, locate all the work places within the geographic area you have defined, then identify a contact person in each place of work. If a Chamber of Commerce exists for the area, you might begin there. Labor unions can also assist you in identifying groups of workers and in providing data on health benefits or services presently in place.

The assessment may focus on the population served by a particular agency, a unit within that agency, a neighborhood, an institution within the community, or the community as a whole. In some cases, an assessment may constitute a research project seeking data to support or reject hypotheses.

If your agency is seeking rural health clinic status in order to qualify for provider reimbursement under the Rural Health Clinics Act, a community assessment is one step in the approval process (16).

In his book, *Community Health Assessment*, Hanchett (17) has developed a tool kit for community health assessment based on general systems theory, which represents one approach. This book identifies the important components, or subsystems, of the system a community represents, tells how to assess those subsystems which are critical to the study, and offers guidelines for identifying relationships and their attributes. An instrument or instruments for assessing the needs of a community could be developed from the material presented.

In doing a needs assessment, Cordes (15) points out that the difference between need and demand should be considered. He also urges that expected outcomes from meeting health care needs be identified as well as measurable indicators of health care needs. He defines needs as services which should be available regardless of economics and demand as an economic concept. The social costs of particular health risks should also be considered in the assessment process and measured so that these data can be considered in setting priorities on health care planning (15).

After the data collection has been completed, data must be organized, tabulated, analyzed, and a report written or prepared in order to share and preserve the information. The report should include purpose and objectives for the community assessment, data collection, findings, and recommendations. From the report you should be able to generate an action plan with measurable outcome criteria.

Model for a Community Assessment

Rationale for Using a Nursing Model

Using a nursing model to structure a community assessment has several advantages. First, it provides a framework not only for the assessment process, but also for the development of a program of intervention based on findings from the assessment. Second, it forms the basis for nursing practice. Third, it is a framework from which to generate research questions as a component of delivery of care. Records for clients can be developed from the model. Protocols for nursing management evolve from the model; evaluation tools to monitor the quality of care and client satisfaction can also be generated through the model.

Ford (18) urges that if we want roles as providers of primary care, we must develop components of health care delivery which are superior to those offered by other health care providers. She emphasizes the need to use "an educative-behavioral model of practice rather than a medical one, if we are practicing nursing." Lytle (19) points out that nurses have only recently begun to produced descriptions of services they can offer to clients. The implication is that we need to do far more documentation to provide data to support our role as health care providers and as a basis for accountability.

Wellness, assessment and interventions, caring, comforting, teaching, counseling, and coordinating are functions Mauksch (20) identifies as appropriate for nurses, and should be part of a nursing model for practice, but are not a major part of the medical model which focuses on illness, diagnosis, treatment, and curing.

Using a model for nursing practice as a framework for a community assessment would, therefore, seem appropriate. The examples that follow demonstrate the use of the model.

Examples of Using a Nursing Model for Community Assessment

The Crisis Nursing Model is presented here as an example of a

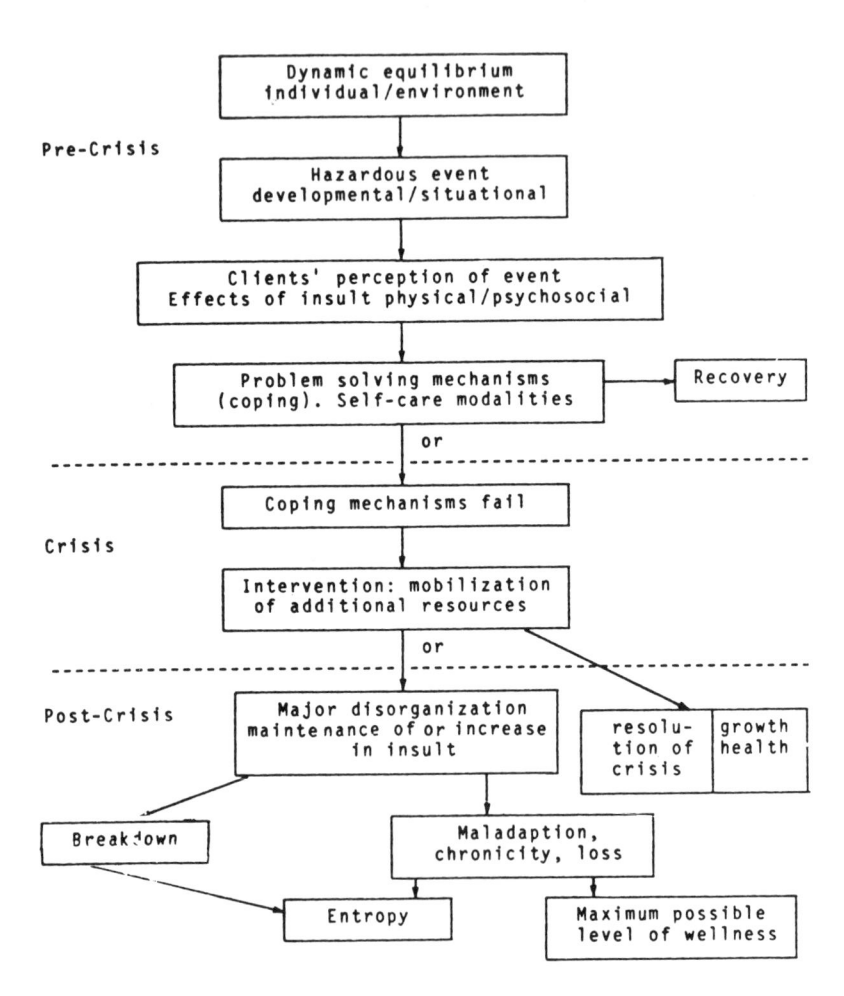

Figure 12.1. Stages of Crisis Theory*

Pre-Crisis

- Dynamic equilibrium individual/environment
- Hazardous event developmental/situational
- Clients' perception of event Effects of insult physical/psychosocial
- Problem solving mechanisms (coping). Self-care modalities → Recovery

or

Crisis

- Coping mechanisms fail
- Intervention: mobilization of additional resources

or

Post-Crisis

- Major disorganization maintenance of or increase in insult → resolution of crisis | growth health
- Breakdown
- Maladaption, chronicity, loss
- Entropy
- Maximum possible level of wellness

*Adapted from University of Connecticut School of Nursing, Storrs, Connecticut

conceptual model for nursing practice upon which a community assessment might be based.

A summary of the four essential components of a model in the context of the crisis nursing model appears in Table 12.1. Stages of the crisis are outlined in Figure 12.1. A complete discussion of crisis model

---

Table 12.1 Essential Components of a Nursing Model: Crisis

INDIVIDUAL (PERSON)
    Physiological
    Psychological
    Social being
    Open system within environment
    Holistic
    Dynamic
    Active role
    Exists on orderly, consistent developmental continuum
    Existence: interrelated balance of external and internal relationships
    Participant: uses problem solving and decision making
ENVIRONMENTAL
    Internal and external forces
    Alters and is altered by individual
HEALTH
    Exists in relation to illness and environment
    Illness: prolonged state of disequilibrium or maladaptation
    Individual's perceptions affect definition of health
    Maintenance of equilibrium and successful coping are indices of health
    Wellness-illness-wellness model
NURSING
    Process based on sciences and humanities
    Augments coping behaviors
    Mobilizes resources
    Intervenes to prevent crisis, restore wellness
    Intervenes in crisis to restore maximum possible level of wellness post-crisis
    Process interactional
    Manipulates external or internal environment to help achieve or maintain higher level of wellness, prevent crisis
    Independent and interdependent functions

is beyond the scope of this book and is unnecessary to the present discussion. A listing is included in the reference list for those interested in a description of the model and its evolution (21).

In basing a community assessment on the Crisis Nursing Model, we must assess the stage of crisis represented by the community. Most communities will be in pre-crisis at the time of the assessment since advanced practice nurses in primary care are most concerned with individuals and communities in pre-crisis. However, assessment may also occur in a crisis situation such as immediately after a natural disaster. Or it may occur post-crisis, e.g., in the aftermath of a crisis such as a riot. Such post-crises assessments resulted in the establishment of neighborhood health centers for primary care after the urban riots of the 1960s and 1992.

At times, there may be an overlap of community assessments conducted by public health (community health) or visiting nurses and nurse practitioners or clinical nurse specialists. Primary care assessments focus on the primary health care needs of individuals, families, and communities whereas public health field studies are broader in scope, encompassing primary, secondary, and tertiary needs of communities as a whole as well as of those who comprise those communities. Clinical nurse specialists may focus their practice on clients needing secondary and/or tertiary intervention (crisis or post-crisis). Any community assessment, therefore, requires that communication with health care providers within the community be studied to determine what assessments have been or are being done. In this way, duplication can be avoided.

Example: Pre-Crisis. The group to be assessed is the population of women over 60 in a New England semi-rural community. The stage of crisis identified is pre-crisis.

1. Elicit the perceptions of those who can help you gather data. These may include the potential target population for services, local health care providers, the director of the senior center, the dean of the school of nursing located in the community, town officials, and social welfare persons.

2. Identify hazardous events, both developmental and situational, which are or may be present. Examples of such hazardous events appear in Table 12.2.

Table 12.2 Hazardous Events

DEVELOPMENTAL (MATURATIONAL)
  Loss of reproductive integrity: menopause, processes of aging
  Loss or threat to intimacy: loss of partner, diminished sexual interest, declining sexual expression
  Loss of relationships: empty nest, death of partner/mate, loss of friends, retirement
  Body image change: processes of aging

SITUATIONAL
  Sexual assault
  Accidents
  Threat to or loss of: independence, mobility
  Threat to or loss of body integrity: processes of aging; chronic conditions in older adults; body image changes: mastectomy, hysterectomy
  Financial loss

---

3. Factors that affect the potential for an optimal level of health must also be identified. These may also be called the resources available, both intrinsic and extrinsic. Table 12.3 lists some which might be identified.

4. Develop tools to collect data on the group targeted for the assessment as well as the resources in the community available to them and the women's own perceptions of their health care needs and their present problem-solving mechanisms.

Findings from the assessment may show that the services needed by the women might be included in an already existing agency, or that new modes of health care delivery should be designed or new services created. An example might be a women's health center staffed by one or more women's health clinical nurse specialists/nurse practitioners located in a community hospital. Psychiatric and community health clinical specialists, gerontologic nurse practitioners, and other advanced practice nurses might be part of an intradisciplinary team.

Example: Post-Crisis. The community to be assessed is a neighborhood in a city. The assessment area is ten blocks long on each side and bordered on one side by a large expressway and on another by railroad

Table 12.3 Factors that Affect Potential for Optimal Level of Wellness

INTRINSIC	EXTRINSIC
Genetics	Socioeconomic status
Nutrition	Resources
Race	financial
Sex	social
	religious
	political
	cultural
	health care
	Education
	Peers
	Family
	Significant others
	Environment
	home
	work
	social
	geographic

lines. The neighborhood is largely residential with a few small commercial establishments, mostly small grocers, package stores, bars, and cafes. Its inhabitants are mostly African-American or recent arrivals from Puerto Rico, and there was a riot less than two months ago which resulted in one death and the gutting of several buildings. Community leaders have identified the lack of available and acceptable health services as one of the precipitating factors.

Thus, the community has recently experienced a crisis, and is now in the post-crisis stage. Beginnings of resolution are identified by community leaders. As a nurse in advanced practice, you are part of a group of health care providers called upon to do a community assessment upon which to develop a plan for neighborhood-based health services.

During the assessment process, it is important to elicit perceptions of both the crisis and the post-crisis state of the neighborhood from those affected and those who may be resources - community leaders, health care providers, and so on.

Hazardous events which may be identified for this community are listed in Table 12.4. Many of these have important implications for nurses as care providers.

Some factors that will affect the potential for the people in the community to obtain an optimal level of wellness are listed in Table 12.5.

In this particular neighborhood, several outcast groups are identified: ethnic minorities, adolescents, single parents, teen parents, and older and aging adults. Some of the hazardous events common to older adults, adolescents, and women are particularly appropriate for nursing management. Examples include challenges of teen and single parenting, chronic disease, obesity, death of spouse/significant others and other losses, and diminishing abilities for activities of daily living. Nurses possess the background to understand the growth and development of all age groups and the skills to assist them.

Table 12.4 Hazardous Events

DEVELOPMENTAL (MATURATIONAL)
  Changing ethnic composition of population in neighborhood
  Deterioration of housing: tenements built 40 or 50 years ago
  Shift in prevalent age groups in population to adolescents and young
     adults and those over 60
  High birth rate, especially to teen population
  Single parent households: women heads of households

SITUATIONAL
  Unemployment rate high due to closing of auto assembly plant
  Construction of 120 units of public housing two years ago
  Completion of expressway cutting neighborhood off from downtown
  Retirement of only family practice doctor in neighborhood
  Riot destroying commmercial block and 15 housing units
  Political climate: cuts in federal spending for health and welfare
     programs

Table 12.5 Factors that Affect Potential for Optimal Level of Wellness

INTRINSIC
Emergence of new community leaders
Community dedication to rebuild grammar school, high school
Three civic/fraternal groups with buildings
Hospital located within three miles of center of neighborhood
Public transportation
Community rooms in public housing projects
Active visiting nurse and public health nursing services in city
One school nurse with primary care preparation
Three active churches in neighborhood
Several vacant buildings in reasonable repair

EXTRINSIC
Federal monies available through H.U.D. for renovation or construction of a neighborhood health center
Eligibility for National Health Service Corps provider(s)
Interest in area health by professional schools in the neighborhood
Plans for a major corporation to locate a division on periphery of target area

Summary

The process of community assessment can be exciting and challenging. In addition to the obvious benefits of identifying underserved or alienated groups of individuals, caseloads may be increased, those not receiving any health care can be identified, populations of clients who have similar problems can be classified, and quality and quantity of care services can be increased.

An understanding of the complexity of events which impact on the health of a community and its potential for an optimal level of wellness can be gained through a more global perspective; the articulation between individuals who are concerned about the health of a community may begin with such an assessment; and the diverse views divulged may generate new ideas for resources to be tapped.

Nurses have an opportunity to define the kind of practice they can be accountable for. A new image of nurses as professional health care providers can emerge. To quote Margaret Walsh, "Nursing . . . is in the process of dynamic change" (22). In order to become independent and interdependent as providers, we must define our scope of practice and delineate the populations whom we may best serve. We need to be able to affect change in our public image, to "facilitate our evolution as the largest and most effective group of health care providers" (22). One way to further this process is to initiate community assessments as one form of market survey in order to identify those for whom we are best prepared to provide health, illness, and wellness care.

REFERENCES

1. Ford, L. (1980). Wellness focus for nursing practice. Unpublished paper presented at Wellness: Focus for the 80s. American Nurses' Association Annual Conference for the Council of Primary Health Care Nurse Practitioners, Philadelphia, Nov. 13-15, 1980.
2. Nursing: A Social Policy Statement. (1980). Kansas City, MO: American Nurses' Association. p. 25.
3. Extending the Scope of Nursing Practice. (1971). Report to the Secretary of Health, Education, and Welfare prepared by the Secretary's Committee to Study Extended roles for Nurses. Washington, DC: Government Printing Office.
4. Wald, L. (1915). The House on Henry Street. New York: Holt, Rinehart & Winston.
5. Dock, L.L. & Stewart, I.M. (1938). A Short History of Nursing. 4th ed. New York: G.P. Putnam's Sons. p. 33.
6. Breckinridge, M. (1952). Wide Neighborhoods. New York: Harper & Brothers.
7. Fuller, L. (1980). Public Health Nursing in Chicago in the 20s, Reminiscences of a Visiting Nurse. Unpublished material.
8. A statement on nurses in primary health care. Primary Care by Nurses: Sphere of Responsibility and Accountability. (1977). Kansas City, MO: American Academy of Nursing. p. 3.

9. Milio, N. (1975). The Care of Health in Communities: Access for Outcasts. New York: Macmillan, p. 57.
10. Bigbee, J.L. (1992). Frontier areas: Opportunities for NPs' primary care services. The Nurse Practitioner 17(9):47-48; 50; 53-54; 57.
11. Nelson-Conley, C.L. (1990). Role development of the clinical nurse specialist within the Indian Health Service. Clinical Nurse Specialist 4(3):142-146.
12. Bowman, R. (1980). Financing for wellness care. Unpublished paper presented at Wellness: Focus for the 80s. American Nurses' Association, Annual Conference for the Council of Primary Health Care Nurse Practitioners, Nov. 13-15, Philadelphia.
13. Ruybal, S.E., Baumens, E. & Fasla, M.J. (1975). Community assessment, an epidemiological approach. Nursing Outlook 23:365-368.
14. Smith, M.C., Barton, J.A. (1992). Technologic enrichment of a community needs assessment. Nursing Outlook 40(1):33-37.
15. Cordes, S.M. (1978). Assessing health care needs: Elements and processes. Family and Community Health 1:1-16.
16. Rural Health Clinic Services. (1979). Washington, DC: Department of Health, Education, and Welfare.
17. Hanchett, E. (1979). Community Health Assessment. New York: John Wiley & Sons.
18. An interview with Loretta Ford. (1975). The Nurse Practitioner 1:9-12.
19. Lytle, N.A., (1977). Jurisdiction of nursing: Areas of control and accountability in delivery of primary health care services. In: Primary Care by Nurses: Sphere of Resonsibility and Accountability. Kansas City, MO: American Academy of Nursing, p. 21.
20. Mauksch, I. (Feb. 28, 1977). Unpublished speech presented at Boston College, Alpha Chi Chapter, Sigma Theta Tau.
21. Hawkins, J.W. (1983). Description, analysis, and evaluation of a developmental model. In: J.A. Thibodeau, Nursing Models: Analysis and Evaluation. Monterey, CA: Wadsworth.
22. Walsh, M.E. (1979). Planning for the future - nursing's role. In: Health Care in the 1980s. Who Provides? Who Plans? Who Pays? New York: National League for Nursing.

Appendixes

Appendix A. Scope of Practice Statements and Role Definitions

Case Management by Nurses, 1992*
The Scope of Nursing Practice, 1987*
Nursing: A Social Policy Statement (1980)*
A Statement on the Scope of **College Health** Nursing Practice, 1992*
Standards and Scope of **Gerontological** Nursing Practice (1987)*
A Statement on the Scope of **High-Risk Perinatal** Nursing Practice, 1980*
A Statement on the Scope of **Home Health** Nursing Practice, 1992*
Standards and Scope of **Hospice** Nursing Practice, 1987*
A Statement of the Scope of **Maternal and Child Health** Nursing Practice (1980)*
A Statement on the Scope of **Medical-Surgical** Nursing Practice (1980)*
The **Obstetric-Gynecologic/Women's Health** Nurse Practitioner. 3rd ed. (1990)**
Scope of Practice for the **Pediatric** Nurse Practitioner (1980)*
The Scope of Practice of the **Primary Health Care** Nurse Practitioner, 1985*
Statement on **Psychiatric and Mental Health** Nursing Practice, 1976*
Rehabilitation Nursing: Scope of Practice; Process and Outcome Criteria for Selected Diagnoses, 1988*

---

* Kansas City, MO: American Nurses Association
** Washington, DC: The Nurses Association of the American College of Obstetricians and Gynecologists (NAACOG)

Appendix B. Resources on Legal and Ethical Aspects, Credentialing, and Certification

State Boards of Nursing. Annual Directory in American Journal of Nursing, issued every April.
Patient's Bill of Rights. Copies from American Hospital Association, 840 N.Lake Shore Dr., Chicago, 60611.
Code for Nurses with Interpretive Statements (1985). Pub. G-56.*
Case Management by Nurses, 1992*
The Scope of Nursing Practice, 1987*
Statement on Psychiatric and Mental Health Nursing Practice, 1976*
Rehabilitation Nursing: Scope of Practice; Process and Outcome Criteria for Selected Diagnoses, 1988*
The Scope of Practice of the Primary Helth Care Nurse Practitioner, 1985*
A Statement on the Scope of High-Risk Perinatal Nursing Practice, 1980*
Standards and Scope of Hospice Nursing Practice, 1987*
A Statement on the Scope of College Health Nursing Practice, 1992*
A Statement on the Scope of Home Health Nursing Practice, 1992*
Credentialing in Nursing: Contemporary Developments and Trends (1987)*
American Association of Occupational Health Nurses, Inc., 50 Lenox Pointe, Atlanta, GA 30324
Center for Credentialing Services, American Nurses Association, 600 Maryland Avenue SW, Suite 100 West, Washington, DC 20024-2571

Advanced Practice Clinical Areas:
Adult nurse practitioner
Adult psychiatric and mental health nursing clinical specialist
Clinical specialist in child and adolescent psychiatric and mental health nursing
Clinical specialist in medical surgical nursing
Clinical specialist in community health nursing
Family nurse practitioner
Gerontological nurse practitioner
Clinical specialist in gerontological nursing
Pediatric nurse practitioner

---
*Order from: American Nurses Association, 600 Maryland Avenue S.W., Suite 100 West, Washington, DC 20024-2571.

(continued)

Appendix B, Continued

School nurse practitioner
Advanced Practice Nursing Administration Area:
Nursing administration, advanced
The National Certification Corporation. 645 N. Michigan Avenue, Suite 1058, Chicago, IL 60611. Certification examinations for:
Ambulatory women's health care nurse
High risk obstetric nurse
Inpatient obstetric nurse
Low risk neonatal nurse
Neonatal intensive care nurse
Neonatal nurse practitioner
Obstetric/gynecologic nurse practitioner
Reproductive endocrinology/infertility nurse
American Association of Neuroscience Nursing, 224 N. Des Plaines, Suite 601, Chicago, IL 60661.
American Association of Nurse Anesthetists, 216 Higgins Road, Park Ridge, IL 60068-5790.
American College of Nurse-Midwives. 1522 K Street, N.W., Suite 1000, Washington, DC 20005.
American Nephrology Nurses Association. N. Woodbury Road, Box 56, Pitman, NJ 08071.
American Society of Ophthalmic Registered Nurses, P.O. Box 193030, San Francisco, CA 94119.
American Urological Association Allied, Inc., 11512 Allecigic Parkway, Richmond, VA 23235.
Association for Practitioners in Infection Control. 505 E Hawley Street, Mundelein, IL 60060.
Emergency Nurses Association, 230 E. Ohio, Suite 600, Chicago, IL 60611.
International Association for Enterostomal Therapy, 2724 La Paz Road #121, Laguna Niguel, CA 92656.
International Society of Nurses in Genetics, 5775 Glenridge Drive, Building A, Suite 150, Atlanta, GA 30328.
Intravenous Nurses Society, Inc., 2 Brighton Street, Belmont, MA 02178.
National Association of Orthopaedic Nurses, Inc., N. Woodbury Road, Box 56, Pitman, NJ 08071.

(continued)

Appendix B, Continued

National Association of Pediatric Nurse Associates and Practitioners. 1101 Kings Highway, Suite 206, Cherry Hill, NJ 08034.
National Association of School Nurses, P.O. Box 1300, Scarborough, ME 04074-1300.
National Nurses Society on Addictions, 5700 Old Orchard Road, 1st floor, Skokie, IL 60077-1057.
Oncology Nursing Society, 501 Holiday Drive, Pittsburgh, PA 15220.

Appendix C. Evaluation Tool for Primary Care with Children*

	POOR	FAIR	GOOD	VERY GOOD
1. Synthesizes knowledge of lifespan's physiological, sociological, psychological factors in primary care delivery				
a. Utilizes the theories of development when providing anticipatory guidance to parents.				
b. Is cognizant of the developmental, physiological, psychological, and sociological factors which necessitate specific planning and management strategies for children.				
2. Demonstrates continuing improvement with well-child assessments.				
a. Is able to conduct a history and physical exam with two children simultaneously.				
b. Is able to identify problems with growth and/or development.				

(continued)

Appendix C. (continued)

	POOR	FAIR	GOOD	VERY GOOD
c. Administers DDST, immunizations, and arranges for lab data with a sense of confidence.				
d. Relates to parent(s) and counsels appropriately re findings during the well-child exam.				
e. Arranges for follow-up appropriately with the help of the preceptor.				
3. Demonstrates continuing improvement in assessing and managing children with a specific problem (walk-ins).				
4. Integrates the responsibility for the continuum of care for a caseload of clients into the broader role of primary care provider.				
a. Utilizes other health personnel when appropriate for communication of plan of care (i.e., social worker, school nurse, etc.)				
5. Evaluates the total role of primary care provider.				
a. By concentrating on well-child visits, demonstrates ability to contact with client at point of entry into the health care system, and provide for follow-up and continuity of care from that point, assessing child within context of family/community.				

(continued)

Appendix C. (Continued)

	POOR	FAIR	GOOD	VERY GOOD
b. Integrates the role of primary care provider as teacher, counselor, and health promotor.				

KEY:
   POOR: Inability to complete the stated objective.
   FAIR: Completes the objective, but requires much supervision.
   GOOD: Completes the objective with minimal supervision or guidance.
   VERY GOOD: Completes the objective independently.

COMMENTS:

---

* Developed by Catherine Collins, RN, MS, and used with permission.

Appendix D. Evaluation Tool for Primary Care with Older Adults*

	POOR	FAIR	GOOD	VERY GOOD

1. Utilizes the Crisis Model of nursing assessing, planning, managing, and evaluating developmental and situational vents.
   a. Demonstrates ability to differentiate pre-crisis and crisis states based on the physical, psychological, and social data gathered on the individual within the framework of his family and community.
   b. Demonstrates ability to differentiate variations of normal from abnormalities during the physical examination/assessment.
   c. Has ability to plan with client as the problem is defined by client's perception of the event.
   d. Helps to facilitate the client's internal resources (present coping mechanisms, nutritional status, activity level, compliance with medications, etc.) and external resources (family, community, agencies available) in management of the present problem. Problem may be a situational (physical, emotional, social) or developmental (i.e., birth, pregnancy, marriage) hazardous event. This includes decreasing the hazardous potential via consultation with an M.D. for management of medical problems, anticipatory guidance, and health counseling.

(continued)

Appendix D. (Continued)

	POOR	FAIR	GOOD	VERY GOOD

e. Demonstrates ability to evaluate effectiveness of management with client at follow-up visits, by re-assessing both client's and provider's perception of the event.

2. Demonstrates increasing knowledge of pharmacological agents (particularly antihypertensive meds) in preventing illness and restoring and maintaining health.

3. Synthesizes the knowledge of lifespan physiological, sociological and psychological factors in delivery of primary care.
   a. Utilizes theories of development in assessing the needs of the elderly.
   b. Utilizes family systems theory in assessing needs of the individual in the context of his/her family environment, and in planning management strategies to meet those needs.

4. Integrates wellness strategies for management within a medical model of care (i.e., exercise prescriptions, focus on diet, and reduction of stress factors).

5. Integrates the responsibility for the continuum of care for a caseload of clients into the broader role of primary care provider.

(continued)

Appendix D. (continued)

	POOR	FAIR	GOOD	VERY GOOD
a. Utilizes other health personnel when appropriate for communication of a plan of care (i.e., social worker, M.D., VNA, rehabilitation agencies, etc.)				
b. Integrates the role of primary care provider as teacher, counselor, and health provider.				
6. Evaluates the total role of primary care provider.				

KEY:
 POOR: Inability to complete the stated objective.
 FAIR: Completes the objective, but requires much supervision.
 GOOD: Completes the objective with minimal supervision or guidance.
 VERY GOOD: Completes the objective independently.

COMMENTS:

---

* Developed by Catherine Collins, RN, MS, and used with permission.

Appendix E. Funding Sources. Publications.

FEDERAL FUNDING SOURCES
Commerce Business Daily
Federal Register
Catalogue of Federal Domestic Assistance
Annual Register of Grant Support
Federal Grants and Contracts Weekly
Health Grants and Contracts Weekly

FOUNDATION FUNDING SOURCES
Foundation Directory and Foundation Grants Index
Annual Register of Grant Supports
Foundation News
State directories of foundations
Academic Research Information System Funding Messenger
The Foundation Grants Index
Source Book Profiles
The Catholic Guide to Foundations

Appendix F. Sources for Information on Grants

American Nurses Foundation, 1101 14th Street NW, Suite 200, Washington, DC 20005.

The Grantsmanship Center, 1031 S. Grand Avenue, Los Angeles, CA 90015.

The Foundation Center, 888 7th Ave., New York, NY 10019.

White, V.: (1983). *Grants. How to Find Out About Them and What to Do Next.* New York: Plenum.

Annual Register of Grant Support. National Register Publishing Company, 3004 Glenview Road, Wilmette, IL 60091.

Catalog of Federal Domestic Assistance. U.S. Office of Management and Budget, Washington, DC 20402.

National Center for Nursing Research. 9000 Rockville Pike, NIH Building 31, Room 5B-03, Bethesda, MD 20892.

Sigma Theta Tau International. 550 West North Street, Indianapolis, IN 46202.

Association for Women's Health, Obstetric, and Neonatal Nurses (formerly NAACOG). 409 12th Street, Washington, DC 20024-2188.

Rubin, M. (1983). *How to Get Money for Research.* Old Westbury, NY: The Feminist Press.

Appendix G. Research References

Annual Review of Nursing Research. (1983, 1984, 1985, 1986, 1987, 1988, 1989, 1990, 1991, 1992, 1993). New York: Springer.

Brink, P.J. & Wood, M.J. (1983). *Basic Steps in Planning Nursing Research, from Question to Proposal.* 2nd ed. Monterey, CA: Wadsworth.

Fawcett, J. & Downs, F.S. (1986). *The Relationship of Theory and Research.* Norwalk, CT: Appleton-Century-Crofts.

Harding, S. (Ed.). (1987). *Feminism & Methodology.* Indianapolis: Indiana University Press.

Krathwohl, D.R. (1977). *How to Prepare a Research Proposal.* 2nd ed. Syracuse, NY: Syracuse University Bookstore.

Locke, L.F., Spirduso, W.W. & Silverman, S.J. (1987). *Proposals That Work.* Newbury Park, CA: Sage.

Morse, J.M. (Ed.) (1991). *Qualitative Nursing Research.* rev. ed. Newbury Park, CA: Sage.

Polit, D. & Hungler B. (1991). *Nursing Research: Principles and Methods.* 4th. ed. Philadelphia: J.B. Lippincott.

Reinharz, S. (1992). *Feminist Methods in Social Research.* New York: Oxford University Press.

Roberts, H. (Ed.). (1981). *Doing Feminist Research.* New York: Routledge.

Sultz, H.A. & Sherwin, F.S. (1981). *Grant Writing for Health Professionals.* Boston: Little, Brown and Company.

Woods, N.F. & Catanzaro, M. (1988). *Nursing Research: Theory and Practice.* St. Louis: C.V. Mosby.

Index

A

Ability and power, 55-57
Admission requirements, lack of unity in, 20-21
Advanced practitioners
  acceptance by other providers, 30-34
  activities (primary) of, 24
  certificate programs for, 20
  certification (see Certification and credentialing for advanced nurses)
  change and, 62-71
  collaboration with other professionals and, 27-30
  collaborative practice and, 149-150
  community assessment and (see Community assessment)
  cost effectiveness of, 155-156
  credentialing of (see Certification and credentialing for advanced nurses)
  employers' ratings of, 31
  employment (see Negotiating an employment contract)
  employment opportunities, new, 150-151
  enlarging client groups, 23
  health care delivery, changing, 62-71
  historical evolution of, 18-22
    certification, 20
    programs for, 20-21
  joint practice and, 28-30
  independent practice and (see Independent practice)
  lack of unity in program requirements, 20-21
  leadership and, 47-48
  legal aspects of role (see Legal aspects of advanced practice)
  marketing services, 23, 157
  medical models and, 10-12
  mentorship and (see Mentorship)
  need for paradigm of empowerment, 52-61
  nontraditional settings and, 23
  nursing models and, 9-17
  power and, 52-61
  powerlessness, roots of, 53-54
  practice settings for, 22-24
  primary activities of, 24
  research (see Research)
  roles (see Roles in advanced practice)
  salaries and, 45-46, 55-56, 156-157
  scope of practice, 25-27

(A, con't)

sex-role stereotyping, 42-51
American College of Nurse Midwives, 21
American Nurses Association (ANA)
   guidelines for advanced practice and, 19, 20, 21
   scope of practice statements and, 25, 26
   state nurse practice acts and, (definition of professional nursing), 73
ANA Congress of Nursing Practice, 19
   definitions of advanced practice and, in 1974, 19-20
ANA Credentialing Center requirement of in 1993 and 1998, 21
ANA Divisions of Practice certification development and, 20
Association of Women's Health, Obstetric, and Neonatal Nurses, 21
   scope of practice statements, 26

B

Breckinridge, Mary, 18
Brown, Esther Lucile, 18

C

Care, boundaries of, and nursing models, 10
Certificate programs, 20
   declining numbers of, 22
Certification and credentialing for advanced nurses, development of, 20
   Appendix B. Resources on legal and ethical aspects, credentialing, and certification, 190-192
   national certification, 76-79
   national credentialing, 80-81
   state certification, 80
Change
   advanced practice nurses as agents of, 64
   bibliography, 71
   concept of, 62-71
   evaluating, 6970
   implementing, 68
   inevitability of, 70
   initiating, 63-64
   reporting change, 70
   theories of, 64-66
      empirical-rational, 65
      normative-re-educative, 65-66
      power-coercive, 66-66
Cleland, Virginia, 44
Clients
   enlarging groups of, 23
Clinical nurse specialists (see also Advanced Practitioners)
   evolution of preparation for role, 21-22
Collaborative practice, 149-150
   "buying into" a practice vs. being a salaried employee, 150
Community assessment, 174-188
   conducting an assessment, 176-178
   formulating a plan for assessment, 176-177
   gathering data, 176-177
   identifying underserved groups, 175-176
   model for community assessment, 179-181
   examples of using a model, 179-

Index

(C, con't)

185
pre-crisis, 182-183
post-crisis, 183-185
Figure 12.1. Stages of crisis theory, 180
Table 12.1. Essential components of a nursing model: Crisis, 181
Table 12.2. Hazardous Events, 183
Table 12.3. Factors that affect potential for optimal level of wellness, 184
Continuous quality improvement, 87-111
bibliography, 109-119
instituting the program, 89-103
audit, 96, 98-100
Table 7.4. Example of audit tool, 99
criteria, standards, norms, 91, 95
Table 7.2. Examples of criteria, 94
defining quality, 89-90
interviews and questionnaires, 103
Table 7.6. Client questionnaire, 104-105
mechanisms, 96-103
Table 7.3. Mechanisms for quality improvement, 97-98
peer review, 100-101
Table 7.5: Peer review worksheet, 102
structure, process, outcome, 90-91
Table 7.1. Measurement domains for quality improvement, 92-93
references, 71-110
standards (listing of), 110-111
Council of Clinical Nurse Specialists, 22
Council of Primary Care Nurse Practitioners (ANA), 22
Credentialing (see Certification and credentialing of advanced nurses)

D

Data
using nursing models to organize and collect, 10

E

Economics of the roles, 141-162
Employment (see Negotiating an employment contract)
Employment opportunities, new, 150-151
Employers' ratings of advanced practitioners, 31

F

Feminist paradigm, need for, 42-51
Funding
Appendix E. Funding sources. Publications, 198
for research, 117

G

Goals
using nursing models to define, 10
initiating change by setting, 63
goal/problem identification, 68
Grants
sources for information on grants. Appendix F, 199

H
Health
 and illness as co-existent states, 12-13
 diagram, "Different conceptions of health," 13
Health care delivery
 changing, 62-71
 advanced practitioners as agents of change, 64
 initiating change, 63-64
 organizational analysis, 64
Health Manpower Act of 1975, 19
Historical evolution of nurse practitioners, 18-22
 certificate programs, 20
 certification, 20
 master's degree programs, 20
Hitchcock, Jane, 151
Hospitals
 nurses' powerlessness and, 53, 55, 56

I
Illness
 and health as co-existent states, 12-13
Independent practice, 141-149
 assessing client population, objective, scope of practice, 142 (see also Community assessment)
 business arrangements, 144-145
 business skills needed, 142-143
 economic uncertainty of, 141-142
 equipment needed, 144
 evaluation and quality improvement, 149
 financial planning, 145-149
 Table 10.1. Start-up costs for independent practice, 146
 Table 10.2. Operating expenses, 147
 Table 10.3. Personal expenses, 148
 Table 10.4. Items that may qualify for deductions, 152
 selecting a site, 143-144
 location, 143
 rent, terms of lease, 143
Influence and power, 54-55

J
Jobs (see Negotiating an employment contract)
Johnson, Dorothy, 19
Joint practice, with other providers, 28-30
 developmental stages of, 29-30

K
Kinlein, Lucille, 22-23, 141, 149, 150

L
Leadership and effect of sex-role stereotyping, 47-48
Legal aspects of advanced practice, 72-86
 Appendix B. Resources on legal and ethical aspects, credentialing, and certification, 190-191
 certification and credentialing
 national certification, 76-79
 national credentialing, 80-81
 state certification, 79-80
 legislation for expanded nursing practice, 74-76
 licensing laws, trends to tighten, 76
 malpractice, issues of, 81-83

Index

nurse practice acts, 73-76
nurse registration statutes, 72
prescription writing, 74-75
references, 83-86

M

Malpractice, issues of, 81-83
Marketing one's services, 23. 157
strategies for, 157
Master's programs
number prior to 1974 and in 1990, 20, 21
rising numbers in 1980s, 22
NLN's 1979 position on, 21
Mayo, Adelaide A., 19
Medical model
danger of nurses using, 11
focus on disease and, 11
nurses and, 10-12
Mentorship, 163-173
alternatives to mentoring, 170
having multiple mentors, 170
paper mentors, 170, 172-173
benefits to the mentee, 166
benefits to the mentor, 165
choosing a mentor, 167-169
avoiding a direct supervisor, 168
defining mentorship, 163-164
disadvantages of mentorship, 166-167
disenchantment, 166
potential conflicts, 166-167
paper mentors, 172-173
references, 171-172
stages of mentoring, 169-170
invitational stage, 169
questioning stage, 169
informational stage, 169
termination, 170
Midwives (see Nurse midwives; also, see Advanced practitioners)
Models, nursing (see Nursing models)

N

National Association of Pediatric Nurse Associates and Practitioners, 21, 25
National Coalition for Action in Politics (N-CAP), 58
National Joint Practice Commission, 28-29
National League for Nursing 1979 position paper on NP education, 21
Negotiating an employment contract, 130-139
bibliography, 139-140
curriculum vitae, 133-134
developing and writing philosophies of nursing and specialty care, 131-132
documents re career, 135
portfolio, developing, 130-136
position description, 134-135
position interview, 136-138
preparing for interview, 137
resume, 132-133
salary, deciding on, 135-136

Nightingale, Florence, 18, 53, 54, and power, 54-58, 59, 63
Nurse clinicians (see also Advanced practitioners)
evolution of preparation for role, 21-22
Nurse midwives (see also Advanced practitioners)
early certificate programs for, 20
guidelines developed for, 21
scope of practice and, 26

Nurse practitioners (see also Advanced practitioners)
  evolution of educational programs for, 20-21
  Nurse Training Act, 19, 59
Nurses (see Advanced practitioners)
Nurses Now (chapter of NOW), 58
Nursing and power (see Power and nursing)
Nursing models, 9-17
  bibliography for, 17
  collecting data and, 10
  defining goals and, 10
  four essential concepts of:
    environment, 12
    health, 12-13
    nursing, 13
    person, 12
  references, 15-16
  medical model and, 10-12
  philosophical issues and, 10
  types of, 10

O
Obstetric-gynecologic NPs
  scope of practice and, 26

P
Pediatric nurse practitioners
  Appendix C. Evaluation tool for primary care with children, 192-194
  acceptance by pediatricians, 30
  scope of practice and, 25, 26
Peplau, Hildegard, 19
Philosophical issues
  nursing models and, 10
Physicians
  acceptance of advanced practitioners, 30-31
  collaboration with, 27
  disease-oriented approach of, 11
  joint practice with nurses, 29-30
  medical vs nursing models, 10-12
  nurses, desire to dictate role of, 44
  sex-role stereotyping and, 44
Power and nursing, 52-61
  ability and power, 55-57
  bibliography, 61
  external resources, utilization of, 58-59
  influence and power, 54-55
  latent power, 54
  powerlessness, roots of, 53-54
  references, 59-61
  strength and power, 57-58
Powerlessness, roots of, 53-54
Practice (see Scope of practice)
Practice, collaborative, 149-150
Practice, independent (see Independent practice)
Practice settings, 22-24
  nontraditional, 23
Primary care (see also Pediatric nurse practitioners)
  Appendix D. Evaluation tool for primary care with older adults, 195-197
PRIMEX program 19
Private practice (see Independent practice)
Programs for advanced practitioners, 20-21
  lack of unity in requirements, 20-21
Prescription writing, 74-75
Psychiatric clinical nurse specialists, 19, 20, 23
Publishing research, 120-124

Index

Q

Quality improvement (see Continuous quality improvement)

R

Reimbursement, third party, 153-155
Research
 bibliography, 128-129
 funding for research, 117
 historical background, 113-114
 identifying researchable problems, 115-116
 impediments to research, 118
 incorporating research into practice, 116-117
 nursing model and, 14
 publishing research, 120-124
 Research reference list, Appendix F, 200
 role of research, 112-129
 translating research into practice, 119-120
 writing up research for publication, 120-124
Roles in advanced practice, 18-41
 interdisciplinary collaboration and, 27-28
 bibliography for, 41
 expanding roles, concept of, 18
 historical evolution of, 18-22
 joint practice and, 28-30
 merging roles between NPs and clinical nurse specialists, 22
 negotiation and, 33-34
 nursing models as guide for, 15
 references for, 34-41
 scope of practice and, 25-27
 sex-role stereotyping, 42-51
 similarities and differences laid out by NP and ANA councils, 22
 socialization into role, 32-34

S

Salaries, 45-46, 55-56, 156-157
 determining before position interview, 135-136
Scope of practice
 statements of, 25-27
 physician statements of, 27
 Appendix A. Scope of practice statements and role definitions, 189
Settings for practice (see Practice settings)
Sex-role stereotyping, 42-51
 bibliography, 50-51
 countering, 57
 dangers of, 43
 leadership, effect on, 47-48
 physicians and, 44
 references, 48-50
 salaries and, 45-47
 self-esteem and, 46, 57

T

Territoriality, conflicts and, 28
Third party reimbursement, 153-155

W

Wald, Lillian, 18, 175
Wellness (see Health)
Women
 depression and, 45
 economics and, 45-46
 need to avoid success, 57
 undervaluation of work by, 45-46
Writing for publication, 120-124